THE OFFSHORE HEALTH HANDBOOK

Prof J. Nelson Norman was formerly Director of the University of Aberdeen's Institute of Environmental and Offshore Medicine, and in 1976 was a member of the Secretary of State's Advisory Group on Health Care Aspects of Industrial Development in the North Sea.

Prof Nelson Norman is now the Director of the Centre for Offshore Health at Robert Gordon's Institute of Technology (RGIT), Aberdeen, and was Honorary Consultant Surgeon to the Grampian Health Board. He is also Consultant to the British Antarctic Survey and was Visiting Professor of Community Medicine to the Memorial University of Newfoundland in Canada. Prof Norman has published over fifty papers in scientific journals and contributed chapters to over twenty books.

John Brebner taught at the Foresterhill College of Nursing in Aberdeen, and joined Prof Nelson Norman as Training Officer at the University of Aberdeen's Institute of Environmental and Offshore Medicine. He is now Assistant Director of the Centre for Offshore Health at RGIT.

THE OFFSHORE HEALTH HANDBOOK

A practical guide to coping with injury and illness

Prof. J. Nelson Norman,
MD, DSc, PhD, FRCS (Glas and Edin),
F Inst Biol, M Inst Pet
*Director, Centre for Offshore Health, RGIT,
Aberdeen*

and

John A. Brebner,
RMN, RGN, HV, Dip Nursing Studies
(Univ of London), M Inst Pet
*Assistant Director, Centre for Offshore
Health, RGIT, Aberdeen*

MARTIN DUNITZ

To Peter Clarke, Principal of RGIT
*whose actions are matched by his vision
in the field of vocational training*

© Prof J. Nelson Norman and John Brebner, 1985
First published in the United Kingdom in 1985
by Martin Dunitz Ltd, 154, Camden High Street,
London NW1 0NE

British Library Cataloguing in Publication Data

Norman, J. Nelson
  The offshore health handbook: a practical
  guide to coping with injury and illness.
  1. First aid in illness and injury
  I. Title   II. Brebner, J.M.T.
  616.02'52   RC87

ISBN 0–906348–80–3

Phototypeset in Sabon by Input Typesetting Ltd, London
Printed and bound in Singapore

CONTENTS

INTRODUCTION

Recent and continuing technological advances in the offshore oil and gas industries have made it possible to extract energy sources from enormously inaccessible places. This, in turn, has created a need for large and increasing numbers of personnel to live and work in extremely remote locations, often associated with intensely hazardous environmental conditions.

The offshore industry requires a high standard of health care for its employees and to achieve this it has been necessary to define a system of medicine designed to cope with the particular problems posed by a remote and dangerous environment—for example, how to manage a casualty suffering from hypothermia or heat stroke when the nearest intensive care unit is many hours away.

The central problem, though, is more logistic than medical and concerns the time and distance which often separate the doctor onshore from his offshore patient. It may take many hours for the doctor to get to the work-site and if the patient happens to be a saturation diver in a pressure chamber at a simulated depth of 600 ft (180 m) the doctor is then faced with a wall of steel which still separates him from the casualty even after he has reached the offshore installation.

In order to provide answers to these types of problems and to help define the components of the system of health care needed, an academic unit was established in Aberdeen in 1976 to consider the medical difficulties that affect people who live and work in remote places subject to hostile environmental conditions. This unit, with which we were both involved, always worked closely with the medical advisers of the oil industry, and the system of health care that emerged was very much a result of the combined efforts of oil company doctors, and physicians in both military and civilian practice.

One of the newly developed basic concepts of offshore health is the need for all offshore personnel to be able to provide correct and immediate care for a colleague who has been injured or who has become acutely ill. In addition to this, the distance factor makes it necessary for offshore workers to be able to describe to the doctor onshore the nature of the problem in sufficient detail to allow him to give precise advice on how to care for the casualty until he can even-

8

tually be brought face to face with a qualified physician.

This book describes the principles needed for good health care in remote workplaces and discusses the particular problems created by the various types of hostile environment. In addition, it gives detailed advice on the immediate action which should be taken for different forms of injury or illness and on the type of information which should be communicated ashore. The advice we give in this book not only forms the basis of many of the courses which have evolved over the years and which are currently offered at our Centre for Offshore Health, in RGIT, at Aberdeen, but also conforms with the British Health and Safety Commission's current recommendations for the training of offshore personnel in health care techniques, which, at the time of writing, are likely to become a legal requirement within the next year or so.

In Aberdeen, we are mainly concerned with offshore installations and with environmental cold, but the same principles of health care apply to all remote work-sites, the fundamental problem being the time and distance which separate the doctor from his patient. There is little basic difference in transportation difficulties across cold seas and hot sands, and from the physiological viewpoint the threats to health posed by intense cold are very similar to those caused by intense heat. The guidelines contained in this book are thus applicable to all remote work-sites—both onshore and offshore—whatever the associated environmental hazard happens to be. In the past years we have been equally happy providing training courses for oil industry personnel in the Arabian Gulf one week and for the personnel of the British Antarctic Survey the next.

Before describing the actual techniques for coping with injuries and illness, we begin the book with two chapters that look at what sort of health problems and risk factors affect the workforce offshore and how offshore health care is now organized.

1. THE PROBLEMS OF OFFSHORE HEALTH

Offshore medicine is the health care available to all those who work offshore. It includes specialized areas of medicine such as the care of divers; it also deals with hygiene and the problems caused by the environment such as extreme heat or cold and the possible presence of toxic gases.

When a rig worker is injured or becomes acutely ill the main problem as far as treatment is concerned is the time and distance which separate him from his doctor. Survival from a serious injury and the quality of survival, for example whether it is accompanied by paralysis, often depends on the skill used in the initial treatment and the speed with which it was given.

Drilling rig in the North Sea. Weather can be extremely severe at times, producing high seas and hazardous working conditions

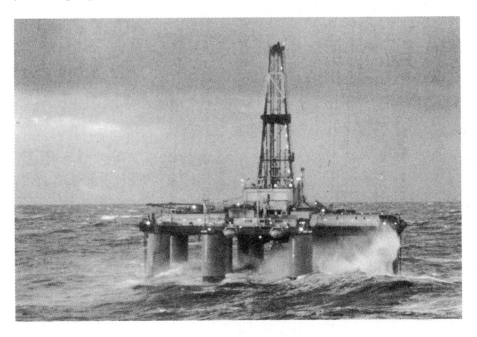

Which injuries and illnesses are most common?

The pattern of injury offshore resembles that of other industrial sites. On fixed installations most injuries occur in relatively young men, and many are the result of falling from a height. Eye injuries are also very common and injuries to hands and arms are common in drillers. On supply boats the injuries tend to occur in an older age group. Crush injuries of the chest and abdomen, with internal damage, result from shifting cargo on rough seas.

Most offshore workers are between twenty and forty years of age and the surveys of accident statistics show that the most common age for serious injury is around thirty years.

Most personnel who become injured or ill offshore are evacuated, because there is no space for caring for the sick for any length of time on a rig. Of those evacuated approximately 35–45 per cent have injuries, and 54–65 per cent have become ill.

The illness and injury statistics for four years on one major operators' installation in the North Sea are shown in the tables opposite. The incidence of serious accidents by occupational groups over a period of time is shown in the diagram below.

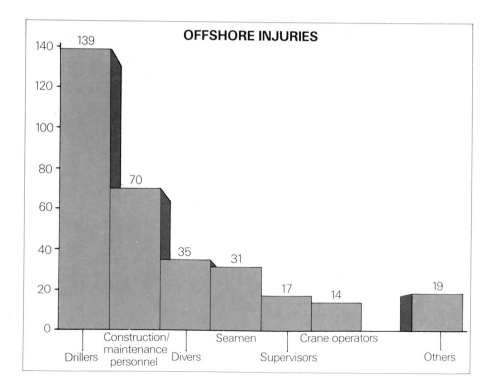

Cause of illness on one platform during four years

	1976	1977	1978	1979
Respiratory	449	214	157	291
Gastrointestinal (e.g. stomach ulcer)	102	53	53	109
Muscles and joints	45	55	21	68
Skin	63	42	39	111
Central nervous system (e.g. stroke)	25	12	15	21
Ear, nose and throat	36	22	17	25
Eyes	9	6	6	40
Dental	22	6	33	39
Genitourinary (e.g. kidney stones)	7	2	12	11
Cardiovascular (e.g. heart attack)	4	2	0	0
	762	414	353	725

Injuries on one platform during four years

	1976	1977	1978	1979
Eye injuries	384	94	80	80
Head and face	54	19	28	19
Hands and arms	194	70	79	89
Feet and legs	107	45	61	59
Back and ribs	45	34	22	21
Scalds and burns	33	9	12	10
Fumes (poisoning)	5	3	4	10
Electric shock	4	0	0	2
	826	274	286	290

Different problems during different phases of development
The normal phases of development of an oil field are:

1. Exploration phase
2. Development phase
3. Production phase.

Opposite: The number of serious accidents by occupation over a period of time.

Exploration phase   In this phase the main activity is drilling to determine whether the geological advice is correct and to discover the presence and the extent of an oil and gas reservoir. Drilling is undoubtedly the most dangerous activity in the oil-related industry, drillers suffering injuries about five times more frequently than any of the other contract workers. Medical facilities on drilling rigs are not usually very sophisticated, though the exploration phase is the most marked for both major and minor injuries. Heavy machinery is used, and hand and head injuries resulting from its use are common. Heavy loads have to be moved from supply boats and workers may be crushed between or under loads. Decks and stairways can become slippery with grease, ice or mud and so falls are common.

Development phase   This follows the decision that the oil field is commercially viable. Preparations are made to install a production platform and to arrange for the oil and gas to be conveyed to the refinery.
   Diving activity is usually added to the drilling and general construction work so there is still potential for a wide variety of serious accidents. During this phase some medical facilities may be available on the rig. In this phase the population is high, there may be overcrowding and the widest variety of medical problems generally occur.

Production phase   This is the stable phase when the population is reduced and the work force becomes an integrated unit. Diving becomes a routine underwater inspection activity with occasional repair procedures. In well-organized production platforms the staff turnover is not high and the work force tends to age gradually in the same jobs. The injury and accident rates fall but there is an increased incidence of the type of illness that generally affects an ageing population, such as peptic ulcers and heart attacks.

The main offshore risk factors

The main factors that contribute to the health and safety risks in the offshore environment are:

1. The environment may be hostile and dangerous (e.g. very hot or cold or noisy).
2. There are constant risks (e.g. helicopter travel, blow-out, gassing and structural failure of platforms).
3. Special workers have special problems (e.g. drillers and divers).

4. The work-site is also where the worker lives.
5. The living accommodation is sometimes overcrowded.
6. It is important to maintain hygiene for the eating and preparing of foods.
7. There may be psychological stress from constant company, long hours and isolation.
8. There are limited leisure facilities.

Hostile environment

Most offshore workings are sited in hostile environmental conditions, for example the intense cold and winds of the northern North Sea or the Beaufort Sea, or the intense heat of the Gulfs of Arabia or Mexico. Water and the high-pressure environment provide further problems for divers. Noise and vibration may also be hazardous. These problems are dealt with in detail in Chapters 7 and 8.

Special risks offshore

Helicopter travel   Offshore installations are normally reached by helicopter, so there is the risk of ditching every time a man goes to work or returns home (see Chapter 6).

Supply boats   Most heavy materials are supplied by sea and one of the serious working hazards is shifting cargo in heavy seas. This may cause crush injuries of the chest and abdomen which are difficult to diagnose accurately and manage in a remote situation.

Structural failure of an offshore installation   Offshore rigs and platforms have been around for some time but those in very deep water such as in the northern North Sea are not more than a decade old and have not yet stood the test of time. Some platforms are built of concrete (for example, the *Brent* and *Beryl* complexes of Shell and Mobil respectively), and some are built of steel (the *Forties* complex of British Petroleum and the *Beatrice* and *Thistle* platforms of Britoil, for instance). Time will tell which design most suits the environment.

So far there have only been two disasters causing great loss of life. In the first the *Alexander Kielland*, a semisubmersible drilling platform was working in the Norwegian sector of the North Sea when one of its three legs sheared off and the whole installation capsized within fifteen minutes. In the second the drilling rig, *Ocean Ranger*, sank off St John's, Newfoundland, in a storm, with total loss of life. It is thought that there was a fault in the stabilizing procedures, but at the time of writing the enquiry findings have not yet been published.

These disasters indicate the vulnerability of offshore installations and show the need for offshore personnel to be trained in survival techniques.

Blow-out occurs when there is a sudden and uncontrolled escape of oil or gas, which usually catches fire. The most disastrous example of an offshore blow-out was when the blow-out preventer was put on upside down in the Ekofisk field in the North Sea. A blow-out occurred, which was fortunately brought under control before too much damage was done. The only casualties were those who left the platform in a panic by lifeboat. The wrong lever was pulled and the lifeboat suddenly fell 150 ft (45 m) to the sea, killing most of those in it. The design of the releasing gear was subsequently changed and greater emphasis was placed on lifeboat training and handling.

Escape of gas   There is always a danger of a sudden escape of gas in any offshore installation and even if it does not cause an explosion or fire, it can rapidly cause death by suffocation.

Hydrogen sulphide is not commonly found in the offshore wells in the North Sea, but it is in the Middle East. Because it is heavier than

One of the most dramatic disasters facing oil industry personnel in remote work-sites is a blow-out.

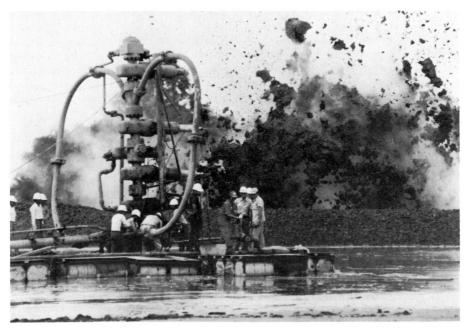

air a substantial and lethal cloud of the gas can soon build up around a structure. Hydrogen sulphide causes respiratory paralysis at concentrations greater than 500 parts per million. Chapter 8 deals with gas poisoning.

Special problems

Divers   Underwater work can be very hard physically and a very high standard of fitness must be maintained by divers if they are to carry out their work safely. They may have to sit in cramped conditions for days, or weeks, until the weather improves and then be required to perform very strenuous tasks. Divers should make use of the recreational facilities on the structure, to keep fit. If divers are present on an installation the rig medic and installation manager must know how to deal with diving-related health problems. These are discussed in Chapter 9.

Drillers   As we have said, the rate of accidents in drillers is five times greater than in any other offshore occupational group. The driller's job requires intense concentration. It is therefore important that he is as free as possible from environmental hazards such as intense heat, cold and fumes, and that he gets plenty of sleep with as little disturbance from noise and vibration as possible. The most common problem for drillers is injury to the hands and arms which can easily get caught in drilling machinery.

Catering staff   All the catering staff must be scrupulous in their standards of personal hygiene, and adequate facilities must be provided to enable them to do so. They require special, periodic medical examination and should, where possible, be provided with their own toilet facilities (see Chapter 10).

Living at the work-site
Space is at a premium on an offshore structure which contains work space, living space and recreational space. Low morale, fatigue and discomfort lead to apathy and carelessness which may ultimately cause accidents.

It is most important for every man on an offshore structure to be aware of the special needs of such a twenty-four-hour community and to help foster the essential community spirit. There can be little doubt that a well-disciplined and happy installation has the most contented work force. This generally means there will be a smaller turnover of workers and consequently a decreased risk of accidents.

Installation managers are aware of this and it is their job to maintain clean, comfortable living quarters with a high quality of food and such recreational and leisure facilities as are possible.

Overcrowded living accommodation

Most installations have no spare living space and in the busy exploration phase there may even be occasions when the same bunk is used for two men on different shifts. Offshore work tends to be dirty, the hours are long and personal hygiene can be difficult to maintain, even though most companies provide an abundance of stewards and facilities such as showers and washing machines. Under these conditions diseases such as scabies may appear, and head and crab lice may proliferate. Overcrowded baths and communal showers lead to ailments such as athlete's foot. These conditions are discussed and explained in Chapter 10. They are serious problems because they can be very difficult to eradicate when they have become established.

When minor ailments like these begin to appear in a closed, overcrowded community they should be regarded as warning signs that the very high standards of hygiene essential to the health of the community are at risk. If a dangerous organism such as dysentery were introduced into the community at that time, it could be disastrous.

Also, under these conditions the morale of the work force is reduced and, as we have said, when that happens the potential for accidents increases.

Eating and preparing food

The provision of good food is essential for the health and morale of the offshore work force. It must be well cooked and presented, and great care must be taken to ensure that it is safe from infection. Chapter 10 deals with the problems of food inspection and handling.

Psychological stress

Though few studies have been carried out on the psychological stresses of offshore workers, our experience of talking to offshore personnel in the North Sea over a decade has shown that, for some, offshore work is not acceptable because it disrupts social and family life. The combination of isolation and the almost overwhelming burden of constant company is also a problem. These men usually opt out quite soon.

On the other hand, recent experience shows an increasing number of offshore personnel who find that the way of life suits them very well. They enjoy the weeks away from home and find that their family life is enhanced by the regular absences. Their work has become routine and enjoyable rather than an adventure. A stable work force is there-fore emerging, and this will do much to reduce the number of accidents.

Leisure facilities
The work shifts are long and often strenuous, leaving little spare time for leisure. Films and video libraries help to allay boredom and some workers use their spare time for private study.

To be safe the offshore worker must be physically fit. But cramped accommodation and good food tend to lead to obesity and lack of fitness. Recently, small gymnasia have been built on several offshore installations. Activities such as weight-lifting and table tennis do not need much space, nor do treadmill jogging machines, which can easily be adjusted to cater for a range of physical abilities.

In summary, although the pattern of injuries offshore resembles that of other onshore industrial sites, there are, as we have seen, special problems and risk factors which make work on oil and gas rigs particu-larly hazardous. And these are compounded by the time and distance separating the casualty from professional medical help. In the next chapter we shall be looking at the way health care teams are organized to cope with offshore emergencies, and explaining the vital role to be played by offshore workers in these situations.

2. HOW OFFSHORE HEALTH CARE IS ORGANIZED

The best solution to the special problems of offshore health seems to be the establishment of a system of medicine which allows for several levels of expertise to function in a coordinated manner, namely, the health care team.

It is important that the rig worker understands how this system operates because he plays a crucial part in it. He may be the only person able to take immediate action when an emergency occurs. When a casualty has been given first aid the rig worker must be able to describe the problem accurately to a doctor onshore, so that high-quality advice can be given. He must then be able to act on instructions from the doctor and carry out the practical manoeuvres suggested by him.

The best care of an injured worker in a remote place is provided as a continuous process from the immediate care on the spot to the treatment in hospital. This can only be achieved with a good network of communications from one level of the health care team to another.

Health care team

The type of people required in a health care team will vary according to the following circumstances:

1. The degree of isolation of the offshore structure and the time taken to obtain help.
2. The size of the offshore population and the type of work being done (e.g. diving, drilling).
3. The communication network available.
4. The methods available for evacuating the casualty and the time it takes to do this.
5. The age and state of fitness of the personnel.
6. The climate in which the work is being undertaken.

Opposite: The offshore and onshore components of the health care team.

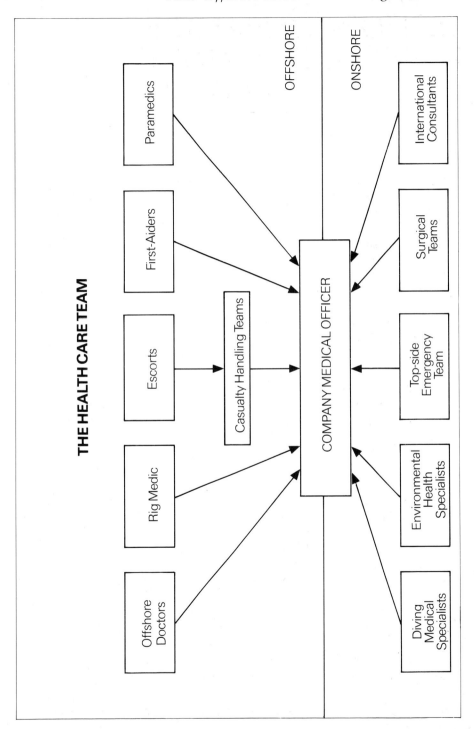

The central figure in the health care team must always be the medical officer of the operating company responsible for the work-site. He is generally based onshore and may be a direct employee of the company, or a medical practitioner retained by the company. He is responsible for the offshore medical personnel, the onshore medical team and coordinating any specialist or hospital facilities required.

The offshore health care team

The primary medical responsibility offshore is held by a doctor, a rig medic or paramedics and first aiders. The number of each depends on the circumstances listed on page 18. There may also be other helpers offshore, such as diving paramedics or life-support escorts. These people generally have other jobs, but are specially trained to give medical help in an emergency.

The offshore doctor   The main advantage in having a doctor offshore is the immediate availability of medical advice and help in an emergency. The presence of a doctor also boosts morale, particularly if the installation is in an isolated place where evacuation may be difficult and take some time. A doctor is the best person to determine the priorities for emergency evacuation of the sick and injured.

In the North Sea, doctors are not normally resident offshore. At the time of writing, the exceptions are the installations *Brent* and *Magnus* which are very remote and are situated close to a large number of adjacent platforms. Although several doctors may be employed to maintain a medical presence offshore, usually only one is resident on an installation at any one time.

Rig medics are generally the main providers of health care on installations. They come from various backgrounds, but are usually either hospital registered nurses, or nurses with military training.

All offshore installations with more than 20 resident personnel have a rig medic, or, in official jargon, offshore sick-berth attendant. If there are more than 200 residents on an installation, two persons with some medical training must be present. Some companies provide two fully trained rig medics, while others provide several people trained in advanced first aid as well as a rig medic.

Paramedics or first aiders   It is becoming more common for a large proportion of offshore personnel to be trained in basic life support or first aid related to their work. Continuing education is given by the company rig medics and at least one day a year is spent practising first aid. This training results in a very high standard of immediate care

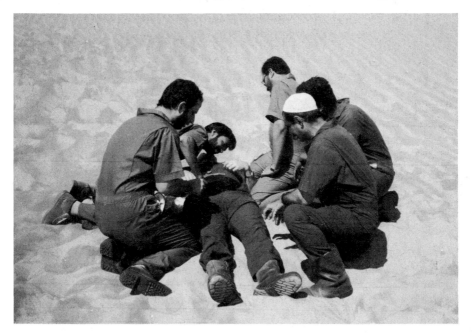

A medical team handling a casualty in the Middle East.

being available. Paramedics are more common in the Gulfs of Mexico and Arabia than in the North Sea.

Life-support escorts are primarily employed for another job on the rig but have had basic first aid training. They have also been given additional training which enables them to escort a serious casualty to shore.

Diving paramedics are divers or supervisors who are trained to look after the special medical problems of divers. Diving paramedics must be able to carry out clinical examinations and be able to report their findings accurately. They must also be capable of carrying out potentially dangerous practical manoeuvres on instruction from a doctor – for example, introducing a needle into the chest to relieve pneumothorax under tension (see Chapter 9). All divers should be trained in relevant first aid. Ideally the supervisor and at least one member of each saturation team should have paramedical training. At the time of writing it is expected that this will become a legal requirement in Britain. Special practical courses are organized for such personnel.

The onshore health care team
This team includes doctors, specialists and environmental health advisors.

Doctors   There must always be a doctor instantly available at the onshore communication centre. This may be a part of the company office, a specially designed onshore health centre or the doctor's home. The doctor should:

1. Be thoroughly familiar with offshore conditions and facilities.
2. Be involved in the health care teaching and inspection.
3. Have discussed emergency procedures with those responsible for health care offshore.
4. Have had some training or experience in teaching appropriate first aid.
5. Know what medical equipment is held offshore.
6. Be familiar with the policies of the company he serves.
7. Be physically fit and prepared to make emergency visits offshore in any weather.

It is essential that the doctor be provided with full information about the casualty so that he can make the best decision and give the best advice to the rig medic or first aider on the spot.

Specialists such as hospital anaesthetists and surgeons should be familiar with the offshore environment and be prepared to travel offshore when necessary.
   There are very few specialists in offshore medicine and diving. Therefore the onshore centre must be able to contact them by telephone, wherever they are in the world. Coordinating networks based in various centres such as Aberdeen in Scotland, Stavanger in Norway and St John's, Newfoundland can help in contacting specialists (see Useful Addresses at the end of this book). It is important that the specialist is given full information on the location of the offshore structure and how far away it is in time and distance. They should also know what communication networks, space and equipment are available. They should also be told about any procedures laid down by the company and, when appropriate, how the procedures relate to the disaster plan for major civil accidents in that area or country.

Environmental health advisers   One of the most important duties of an independent environmental health adviser is to liaise between the offshore installation, on behalf of the operating company's medical department and the public health authorities onshore.

In Britain this liaison activity was established in 1980 by the oil industry when the medical subcommittee of the United Kingdom Offshore Operators' Association (UKOOA) published environmental health guidelines. These have been invaluable in the North Sea and have formed the basis of guidelines used in other parts of the world.

The environmental health adviser is mainly responsible for the standards of food handling and hygiene on an offshore installation and for advising on the management of an outbreak of infection offshore (see Chapter 10). He must visit the offshore structures regularly and should build up a good relationship with the management there. The onshore health authorities are very interested in the risks of infection offshore because infected people may have to be evacuated into the onshore community, so the health adviser also has to keep them informed.

Training rig workers in basic life support

There are two important components to basic life support:

1. Basic training in emergency care and resuscitation (see Chapters 3 and 4)
2. Training in providing an accurate description of the problem to a doctor so that he can give advice on further action (see pages 52–4).

There is no doubt that the quality of the advice given by the onshore doctor is directly related to the completeness and relevance of the information he is given from the offshore installation.

Panic in early communications must be avoided. An extra five minutes taken to assess the situation properly can save hours later or even the patient's life. It does not save time to ask for a doctor to be sent in a hurry while an assessment of the casualty is being made. This may result in the wrong doctor, with the wrong equipment being sent off in the only helicopter available. For example, a casualty with a crushed chest may need the attention of an anaesthetist with a ventilator before he can safely be transferred ashore. Similarly, a man caught in machinery or badly burned may require the help of a surgeon rather than a general doctor.

Even if no specialized help can come for several days a great deal can be done to help the casualty if his colleagues are trained in basic life support and are assisted by a doctor through a good system of communication. This book is based on the courses we run at Aberdeen for training rig workers in basic life support.

Communications

A first-class system of communications is very important in offshore medicine. There should be a direct link between whoever is managing the case offshore (normally a rig medic) and the doctor onshore.

Any communication by voice should always be followed by an exchange of telexes to prevent misunderstandings. Communicating by telex gives thinking time to both parties, allows for the careful formation of the message, helps to eliminate ambiguity and provides a permanent record of the management of the case for future analysis and reference.

There are occasions, though, when medical discussions which can be relayed by telex are difficult to transmit initially by voice. Problems with radio communication include poor quality of transmission, the degree of privacy of the conversation and whether the participants in the conversation know each other well enough to be relaxed.

It cannot be overemphasized that the medical link between the man managing the casualty offshore and the onshore doctor supporting him must, if possible, be direct.

Communicating with the doctor

It is very important that the doctor is given relevant, accurate information about the casualty. He can then decide what treatment is best for the casualty. For example, if he is asked about a man with a severe headache and given no more information, the doctor may tell the first aider to give the patient two aspirins and report back in the morning. That would be the correct decision if the headache resulted from eye strain or fatigue but it may cost a young man his life if the headache is caused by a slow internal haemorrhage from a blood vessel in his head. Such a disaster could be prevented by sending everyone who has a headache ashore, but each time this is done the emergency helicopter costs would be roughly equivalent to at least one year's salary for a rig worker.

Another example of bad communication occurred one winter morning in 1982 when there was a call for a doctor from a ship in the northern North Sea because a man had been shot. No other relevant details were given. In atrocious weather conditions a doctor, a very experienced rig medic and four others took off in a helicopter on an errand of mercy. The helicopter ditched and they were all killed, while the shot man was little the worse for his experience having only sustained a trivial air-hose injury.

To help prevent such misunderstandings, it is vital to practise communication techniques. A useful check-list of points to remember is given on page 54.

Communication with saturation divers
This is a special and more difficult problem because the sick diver and his attendants are locked in a pressure chamber, and the helium in the breathing mixture distorts the voice. The chain of communication will be longer because more people are involved, and so even greater care must be taken to report everything accurately. See page 178 for more details about communicating with divers.

Future developments
Medical conferencing with slo-scan television and telemedicine via satellite systems is already in limited use but may become widely employed in offshore health care over the next few years. When this technology is fully developed it should be possible for medical personnel onshore to monitor the heart's activity by means of electro-cardiogram (ECG) tracings, and to see X-ray pictures and even the patient on a television screen. Much of this technology was originally developed for space exploration.

Medical examination

One of the most valuable medical contributions to health and safety offshore is the pre-employment and repeat medical examination. This determines whether a man is fit to work offshore, in a remote environment potentially isolated from qualified medical assistance. It must be realized that if serious illness develops on an offshore installation a long time may pass before anything can be done about it. An emergency evacuation costs a great deal of money and lives may be put at risk in attempting to bring medical aid to someone who has become injured or ill.

Offshore work schedules may be long and arduous and therefore both physical and mental ability must be carefully assessed. Most offshore installations have numerous stairways and ladders and physical stamina and agility are required to negotiate them. There is no light work in the sense used onshore. The medical examiner must always assess whether a potential offshore worker will perform satisfactorily in an emergency without putting himself or his colleagues at risk.

It has now become standard practice in the North Sea for all contracting companies to assume medical standards similar to those of the operating company which employs them. This has done much to raise the standard of health in offshore workers. Recently the operating companies in British waters came together to produce a list of the minimum standards of fitness in offshore workers. These examinations may be carried out by doctors in other parts of the country or in

Some probable grounds for disqualification at a medical examination

1. Blindness in one eye, or marked defect of vision. Eye diseases such as cataract, trachoma or glaucoma.

2. Menières disease, chronic ear infection and marked hearing loss.

3. Advanced gum disease or severe tooth decay.

4. Gastrointestinal disease such as peptic ulcer, gastritis, ulcerative colitis, etc, and recurrent disease of the gall bladder or liver.

5. Piles causing symptoms; fistulae, colostomy, pilo nidal cysts.

6. Hernia.

7. Long-term kidney disease, kidney stones, prostrate disease. Bed-wetting (present or recent past).

8. Venereal disease.

9. Disease of the testicles.

10. Markedly enlarged or infected tonsils.

11. Lung disease such as: acute tuberculosis, asthma, chronic bronchitis, bronchiectasis, emphysema, pneumothorax.

12. Cardiovascular disease such as a congenital heart condition, high blood pressure, hardening of the arteries, angina or history of heart attacks.

13. Diseases of blood vessels: severe varicose veins (with or without varicose ulcers), peripheral arterial disease.

14. Blood disorders.

15. Partial or full loss of any extremity sufficient in the examiner's opinion to impair full performance of duty.

16. Deformities of joints and limited neck movement due to arthritis, which affects mobility, dexterity and causes pain. Gross obesity.

17. Recent injuries that may lead to progressive disabilities, for example, back injuries, skull fractures.

18. Any organic or progressive neurological or neuro-muscular disease, including multiple sclerosis, muscular dystrophies, epilepsy, any bouts of loss of consciousness and severe migraine.

19. Severe skin disease, including fungus infections, scabies, etc, and psoriasis.

20. Mental illness, personality disorders, emotional immaturity, schizophrenia, depression.

21. History of alcoholism or drug abuse.

22. Evidence of malignant disease at present or in the past five years.

23. Glandular conditions such as diabetes, thyroid disorders, etc.

24. Those on drug treatment with anticonvulsants, hypotensive agents, anticoagulants, cytotoxic agents, insulin, steroids, antiischaemic drugs and tranquilizers.

foreign countries but the operating company normally reserves the right for its own medical advisors to make a final decision about the medical fitness of any individual. These medical examinations are usually carried out at 3-year intervals up to the age of 40 years, every 2 years between the ages of 40 and 50 years and annually over the age of 50 years. A similar medical examination system is being introduced in Canada's eastern seaboard.

So far we have examined in general terms the main health and safety problems that face the worker offshore, and the part he plays in the health care structure that exists to cope with these situations. The chapters that follow explain in detail the practical procedures for dealing with injury and illness on site. First we look at emergency life-saving techniques – all of which are essential for every offshore worker to know.

Opposite: A list of some of the conditions likely to disqualify a potential offshore worker on medical grounds. The person may be re-employed if the problem is corrected.

3. EMERGENCY LIFE-SAVING TECHNIQUES

The action taken in the early stages of a serious injury or illness will often determine the ultimate outcome. Lack of knowledge of the correct procedures to adopt leads to fear and panic for all involved, which is dangerous. This is less likely to happen if the worker helping the victim has the basic know-how on which to base his actions. Even medically qualified personnel may become confused by an element of panic when dealing with serious injury. It is vital therefore that the techniques of life preservation and first aid should be so well known and practised that the immediate response of helpers on the spot will be nearly automatic. This applies to all workers in an offshore installation, whether primarily involved in medical care or not.

This book is concerned with the immediate care of injury and illness to cover the interval of time that will elapse before nursing or medical help is available. The overall term for these skills is basic life support.

Basic life support

The aims of basic life support are to administer immediate treatment and to transport a live patient to hospital without his condition worsening on the way. This is done by:

- Preserving life
- Preventing worsening
- Promoting recovery.

Preserving life

The techniques of life preservation are the subject of this chapter. It is important to remember that the life of the first aider must be preserved as well as that of the casualty. For example, if a man collapses when he is working in an area containing hydrogen sulphide and a colleague rushes to remove him from the dangerous area without using breathing equipment, two deaths may occur instead of one (see Chapter 8). Trying to help a man who has been electrocuted and is still in contact with the electric current, without first switching off the electricity supply, might also cause two deaths instead of one. In both cases a quick assessment of the situation before acting would have preserved life. The immediate actions necessary to preserve the casualty's life are discussed below.

Preventing worsening

When sudden and serious injuries occur it is natural to want to do. something to help, but clumsy and careless handling of a casualty may make the injury worse. In the case of a back injury, for instance, clumsy handling may convert a simple fracture of the spine into a nerve injury, resulting in permanent paralysis. Unless the casualty is in immediate danger and urgent action is essential it is best to plan carefully and slowly the steps which must be taken to help him. While that is being done you should reassure the casualty and protect him from whatever is causing his injury. It is just as important to know what not to do, as it is to know what should be done. In many cases it is better, but more difficult, to do nothing than to do something which might make the injury worse.

Chapter 5 gives details on how to handle a casualty.

Promoting recovery

In most cases this begins with appropriate first aid at the scene of the accident, after the emergency life-saving procedures have been performed. For example, giving oxygen to a patient whose chest has been badly injured may promote his recovery before transport to hospital. The next chapter gives detailed instructions on first aid for the types of injures most commonly sustained offshore.

ABC of life support

The body consists of a mass of individual cells, and the supply of oxygen to these cells is vital to the body's survival. The brain cells suffer permanent damage or death if they are deprived of oxygen for more than three minutes. If a casualty dies it is usually because there have been problems with the following:

- Airway
- Breathing
- Circulation.

It is therefore essential to check that these three systems are functioning correctly, particularly in an unconscious casualty. Anything which prevents oxygen reaching the blood and being circulated to the cells, by the pumping action of the heart, is likely to result in death in a few minutes. These three vital checks can conveniently be remembered as the ABC of basic life support.

Airway

The airway must be kept clear. If it is blocked, oxygen cannot be transferred from the air through the lungs and into the blood. The airway may be blocked, for example, by a piece of meat that has gone down the wrong way or by blood from an injury, or by vomit. Alternatively when an unconscious casualty lies on his back the muscles supporting the tongue become slack and the tongue will fall back, obstructing his airway. Techniques for keeping the airway clear and removing foreign bodies from it are described opposite and illustrated on page 32.

Breathing

Check that the casualty is breathing. This is sometimes very difficult to determine, especially if the casualty is unconscious, the weather is bad, the environment noisy, or if the casualty is wearing heavy clothing. The only effective way to check whether a casualty is breathing is to place your ear close to his nose. If he is breathing it may be possible to hear his breath sounds and to feel the movement of his breath on the side of your face. If you are still in doubt whether the casualty is breathing or not, begin artificial respiration at once (see later in this chapter). Giving artificial respiration to a man who is still breathing will do no harm.

The rate and depth of breathing are controlled by the brain sending signals to the chest wall. Breathing usually stops because of the damage to the centre in the brain which controls breathing. This may result from lack of oxygen due to one of the following three factors.

- The airway is blocked
- The oxygen cannot reach the lungs (e.g. in drowning)
- The oxygen cannot be circulated to the brain (e.g. in a heart attack).

Circulation

If you are sure that spontaneous breathing is still taking place you can assume that the heart has not stopped beating. But if the casualty is unconscious and not breathing, it is necessary to find out whether his heart is beating. This is done by feeling the carotid pulse in the neck (see illustration on page 37). If the heart stops, the blood with its supply of oxygen cannot be pumped to the body cells. It is then necessary to provide oxygen by artificial respiration and to combine this with external heart compression, which pumps the oxygenated blood to the cells (see illustrations on page 38).

First action

If you are the first man on the scene of an accident, it is essential not to panic, but to act in a calm, controlled way. To be able to do this, the immediate actions of basic life support must be practised over and over again so that when the occasion arises to use them they have become automatic – as automatic as ABC.

First of all determine whether the casualty is conscious. If he is conscious and able to speak you can assume his airway is clear and his heart is beating. If he cannot speak he may be choking and you should follow the procedure on page 40. Once you have made sure there are no problems with his airway or circulation, any heavy bleeding or fractures must be dealt with (see pages 42–5 and Chapter 4).

If the casualty is unconscious, send for medical help and begin the ABC of basic life support at once, as described below.

Mouth-to-mouth resuscitation
This sequence of actions should be practised with a manikin on several occasions so that it becomes automatic (see illustrations overleaf).

1. Check the airway is clear by scooping your fingers into the mouth to remove any obstruction, such as foodstuff, vomit or dental plates. Small, partial plate dentures are more likely to cause trouble than full sets of dentures.
2. Place your ear close to the casualty's nose to feel and hear him taking breath in and out.
3. If you cannot feel or hear the casualty breathing then extend his neck, because the windpipe may have been obstructed by the tongue falling back over it. Listen again. If you still cannot detect breathing or if there is any doubt, begin artificial respiration immediately.
4. Keep his head extended to maintain an open airway. The most convenient position for artificial respiration is to kneel beside the casualty's head, to place one hand below his neck and to use the other to pinch his nose shut.
5. Take a deep breath in and place your lips around the casualty's. Breathe your air sharply and evenly into his mouth.
6. To begin with, give four breaths in quick succession. This completely inflates the casualty's lungs and provides them with a reservoir of oxygen to work with.

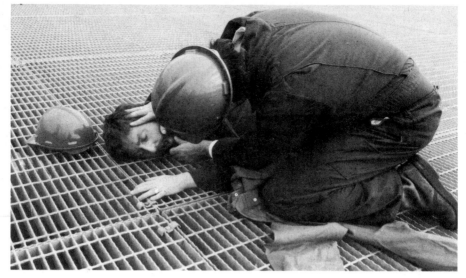

1. **Clearing the airway**   Open the mouth by pulling down on the lower jaw. Clear the mouth with a sweeping motion of the index finger.

2. **Opening the airway**   Open the airway by tilting the head backwards and supporting the neck. This moves the tongue forward with the jaw, preventing it from obstructing the windpipe.

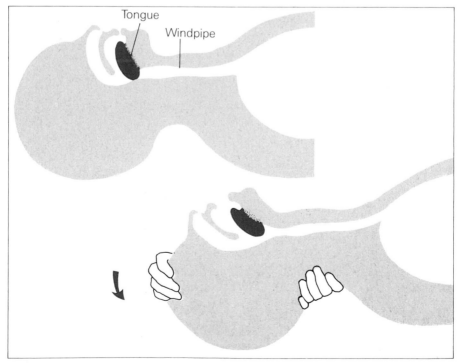

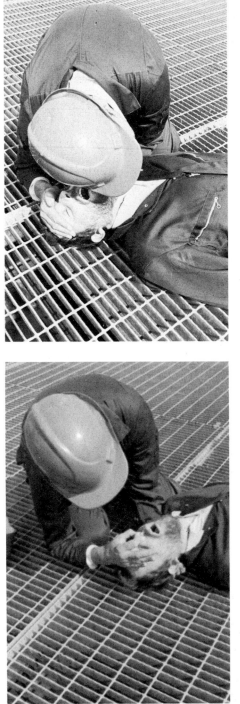

3. **Checking breathing** Look for the rise and fall of the chest. Listen for air coming from the nose and mouth. Feel the exhaled air on your cheek.

4. **Mouth-to-mouth resuscitation** Kneel beside the casualty's head. Open his airway by tilting his head back and holding his neck straight. Pinch his nose to prevent air escaping. Open your own mouth wide to get a good seal around the casualty's lips and blow air into the casualty's mouth to fill his lungs.

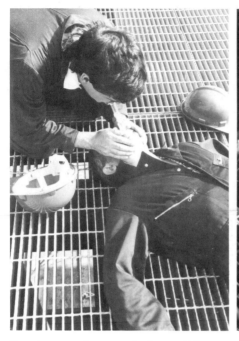
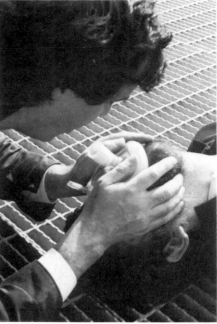

Brookes tube technique When blowing air in through a Brookes tube, position yourself behind the casualty's head and look down over the chest so that you can see the rise and fall of his chest as his lungs fill and empty.

Laerdal mask technique Open the airway by pulling back on the jaw bone. Place the mask flat against the face to get an airtight seal, and blow air in through the tube attached to the mask.

7. Next determine whether the carotid pulse is beating in the neck (see illustrations on page 37).
8. If the carotid pulse is not beating, begin external heart compression (see pages 35–9).
9. If the carotid pulse is beating continue with artificial respiration but reduce the rate to one breath every four seconds.
10. Continue artificial respiration until medical help arrives or the casualty starts breathing spontaneously. A rate of fourteen to eighteen breaths per minute or one every four seconds is sufficient. If you breathe faster than this you will become giddy and may faint.

If there is considerable damage to the casualty's face or if you find the idea of mouth-to-mouth breathing distasteful, other methods of artificial respiration are available. These are commonly held in standard

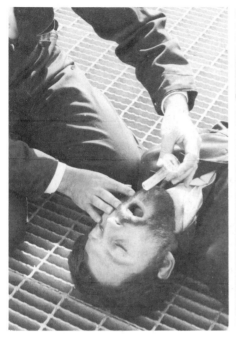 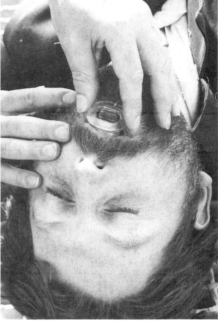

Guedel airway insertion. It is a good idea to insert a Guedel airway into an unconscious casualty to prevent obstruction of his windpipe.
1. Insert the Guedel airway over the tongue with the tube pointing upwards so that the tongue is not pushed down the throat.

2. When the tip of the guedel reaches the back of the tongue, gently rotate the tube 180° and it will slide smoothly into the casualty's airway.

first aid boxes and include the Brookes tube and the Laerdal mask (see illustrations opposite).

External heart compression

What it does The heart is made up of four chambers bound by muscle. When that muscle contracts the volume of these chambers becomes smaller and the blood contained in them is thus pushed onwards. The blood can only move in one direction because at the entrance and exit of each chamber there is a system of one-way, non-return valves.

The heart lies between the breast bone and the back bone; and these are attached to each other by the ribs which are flexible. If the heart stops for any reason it is possible to compress it between these two large bony structures. This reduces the volume of the blood chambers, pushing the blood contained in them forwards. If external heart compression is performed efficiently, a pulse can be felt in the neck with each compression. Heart compression should be given at the same rate as the pulse (eighty times a minute). It will not help the casualty, though, unless the blood which is being circulated to the cells contains oxygen. It is therefore important that an adequate supply of oxygen is maintained by mouth-to-mouth resuscitation, as previously described. This will also ensure that oxygen is supplied to the heart muscle. Restoring the oxygen supply to the heart may be sufficient to restore the heart's normal rhythm of contraction.

The importance of excellent technique   If the heart compression technique is excellent and precise the circulation will be approximately 20 per cent as efficient as if the heart was functioning normally on its own. There is therefore little room for error and it is essential that a precise and excellent technique is learned and maintained. The basic heart compression technique, which is easy to acquire, should be learned from professionals at a good first aid course and maintained by practice at least once a year.

When to start external heart compression   External heart compression should be started as soon as you are sure the heart has stopped beating. Harm can be caused if heart compression is carried out when the heart is still beating. Therefore you must ensure that the heart has indeed stopped beating. Remember:

1. If the casualty is conscious the heart has not stopped beating.
2. If the casualty is breathing the heart has not stopped beating.
3. It may be difficult to feel a pulse at the wrist, therefore check the presence or absence of the carotid pulse in the neck.

How to do external heart compression   When you reach step 7 in the resuscitation procedure for the unconscious casualty (see page 34) you will have determined that he is not breathing, given four lung inflations, and felt for the presence or absence of the carotid pulse in the neck. If the carotid pulse is not felt, begin external heart compression (see illustrations on page 38).

1. Kneel at the casualty's side, close to his chest and in as comfortable a position as possible.
2. Place the heel of one hand over the lower part of the breast bone, two finger breadths above the notch at the bottom junction of the rib cage. Place the heel of the other hand over the first hand and entwine your fingers, keeping them off the chest.

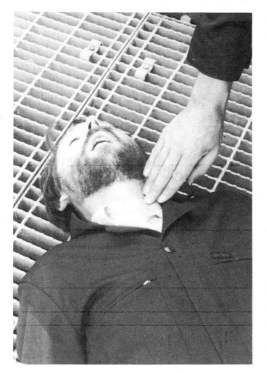

Checking the carotid pulse Place your fingers in the groove between the muscles on the side of the windpipe. Push down firmly to feel the pulse, as the artery may be well covered with muscle.

3. Your shoulders should be in line with the casualty's breast bone and vertically above it. Now it is possible, almost passively, to allow the weight of your body to be transmitted through your straight vertical arms to compress the casualty's heart.
4. This position helps you to carry out heart compression with the greatest comfort and least exertion, allowing you to continue for a longer period of time.
5. With your arms straight, squeeze steadily downwards for about 1½ in (4 cm) and immediately release the pressure. Repeat this movement at a rate of about eighty times per minute.

One first aider should give fifteen heart compressions at this rate followed by two lung inflations and continue at that ratio. The compressions should be stopped every two minutes to check whether the carotid pulse in the neck has returned. If there is still no pulse, continue heart compression. If the pulse has returned, external heart compression should be stopped.

Two first aiders should give five heart compressions followed by one lung inflation and continue at that ratio. The rate of the compression given by the first aider should be sixty compressions per minute because

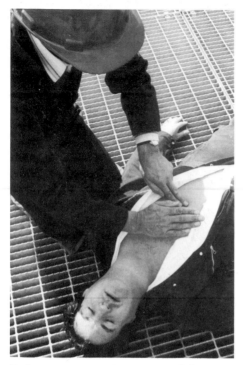

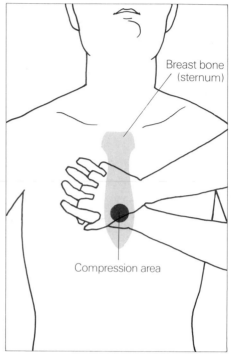

Before commencing external heart compression, lie the casualty on his back on a firm surface. The correct hand position is achieved by finding the top of the V-shaped bone that forms the bottom of the rib cage. Position the heel of one hand two finger breadths above the V-shaped bone so it covers the lower third of the breast bone.

The correct hand position on the breast bone (sternum) for external heart compression.

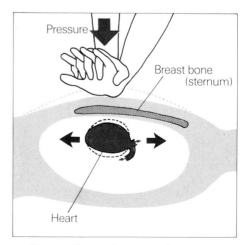

By exerting a downward pressure on the breast bone the heart will be compressed and expel blood.

there will be no pause for lung inflation. The lung inflation carried out by the second first aider should be timed to take place while the hands of the first aider giving heart compression are on the upward movement.

The most experienced first aider should initially control the lung inflation because this is the vitally important part of the operation. He can also feel the carotid pulse to determine whether the heart compressions are adequate. Every two minutes the heart compressions should be stopped to determine whether the pulse has returned.

How long should resuscitation continue?

Heart compression combined with mouth-to-mouth respiration is an extremely tiring procedure and the length of time it can be carried on for will often be determined by the strength of the available first aiders. If you have a good reason for beginning resuscitation, you need a good reason for stopping it. Casualties have recovered after long periods of heart compression, so it should be continued until:

- The patient recovers
- He is pronounced dead by a doctor
- The first aiders are exhausted
- A medically qualified person advises that resuscitation should stop.

Likelihood of success

If breathing has stopped and the heart is still beating the heart will not stop as long as a good supply of oxygen can be provided by mouth-to-mouth respiration. In these circumstances there is a high possibility that resuscitation will be successful. But if the heart and breathing have both stopped then the chances of success are less, because the work of both the heart and the lungs has to be performed artificially.

Casualty handling teams

In very hot climates it is not possible to carry out effective heart compressions for more than a few minutes in the open. In these situations it is important to have a large number of trained first aiders who have practised the technique of taking over either heart compression or lung inflation from colleagues without interfering with the ratio of the resuscitation procedure.

Ideally, this taking-over procedure should be practised in all parts of the world by casualty handling teams specially designated among the offshore work force. These teams are becoming more common; at the time of writing there are forty to fifty operating companies working in the North Sea and most have organized casualty handling teams.

But at present there are few offshore casualty handling teams elsewhere in the world. The availability of a casualty handling team, used to working as a team both for resuscitation and lifting procedures (see Chapter 5) ensures more effective care of casualties. The large numbers of offshore workers trained in basic life support by the oil industry makes this possible, but regular practice of the techniques is essential.

Specific conditions where resuscitation may be necessary

Choking

This occurs when a foreign body – usually food – gets stuck in the windpipe. The casualty tries to cough and is unable to speak. The emergency procedure to adopt is as follows (see Heimlich technique opposite):

1. Ask the casualty: 'Are you choking?' If he is, he will nod.
2. With his head down give him four sharp blows between the shoulder blades.
3. If these do not dislodge the object, stand behind the casualty and put your arms round his body (Heimlich standing).
4. Make a fist with one hand and place it firmly in the soft space between the lower end of the breast bone and the navel. Cup the other hand over this one.
5. Give a hard sharp thrust upwards and inwards.
6. If the casualty is lying down turn him on his back. Kneel across his thighs and apply pressure with the heels of your hands just below his breast bone (Heimlich lying).
7. Repeat until the foreign body is dislodged.
8. You should never attempt to puncture the casualty's windpipe with a sharp instrument. This is far less likely to be successful than the method described above and can cause death in unskilled hands.

Choking (*opposite*)

1. The airway may become blocked if a foreign body such as food becomes lodged in the windpipe instead of continuing down the oesophagus into the stomach.

2. **Heimlich technique (standing)**   Place a clenched first, thumb side facing in, just above the waistline. Place the other hand over the fist and squeeze sharply inwards and upwards under the rib cage.

3. **Heimlich technique (lying)**   Turn the casualty onto his back with his head to one side. Straddle across the casualty's thighs. Place the heel of your hand just above the waistline and position the other hand over the top. Squeeze sharply inwards and upwards under the rib cage.

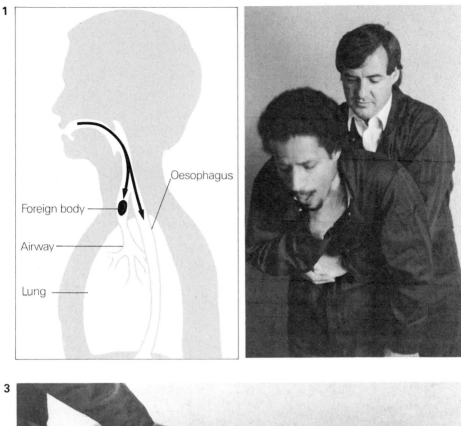

Oesophagus

Foreign body

Airway

Lung

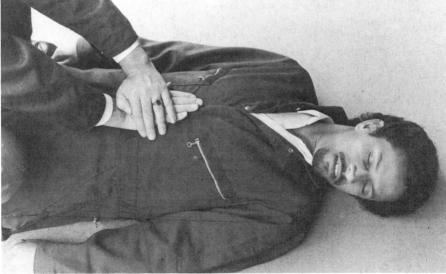

Heart attack

Although the rig population is fitter than the general population heart attacks are not uncommon (see table in Chapter 1). The heart attack victim generally complains of a severe crushing chest pain and breathlessness. The pain may radiate down an arm or up to the jaws.

Heart attacks are commonly caused by a clot forming in one of the arteries which supplies the heart muscle with oxygen. The muscle beyond the clot dies. If the blocked artery supplies a large part of the heart, recovery is unlikely, but if it supplies a small part, recovery is quite possible. Sometimes the whole system is thrown into confusion when a small artery is blocked causing the heart to stop. This is the type of case where you can save the casualty's life if you are able to take over his heart function using external heart compression until his heart begins beating of its own accord again. If you suspect a heart attack and the casualty is conscious:

1. Keep him calm and do not allow him to exert himself.
2. Reassure him and arrange his evacuation to hospital.
3. Keep a close watch on his breathing and pulse rate and be prepared to begin resuscitation if necessary (see previously in this chapter).

Bleeding

When you have attended to the casualty's airway, breathing and circulation, the next priority is to control any severe bleeding. Bleeding varies greatly in severity and nature depending upon the size and type of blood vessel severed and the associated injury.

Bleeding from arteries

Oxygenated blood is carried from the heart to the organs and cells of the body by a system of arteries. These are fairly thick-walled vessels which are lined by muscle and elastic tissue. Arteries have thick walls because the blood is under fairly high pressure when it leaves the heart. Each time the heart contracts, approximately 2½ fl oz (70 ml) of blood are pushed into the circulation and the arteries expand momentarily to accommodate it. This expansion movement is transmitted along the arteries and can be felt as the pulse. When an artery is severed the blood comes out at high pressure, is bright red and spurts in time with the heartbeat.

Control of bleeding from arteries   When blood vessels are severed the natural body mechanism to prevent loss of blood is the formation of a blood clot to block the hole. But when an artery is severed the blood spurts out under high pressure which hinders the formation of a clot. To stop bleeding from an artery, pressure must be applied to the bleeding point. This pressure has to be maintained until the blood, which has now stopped flowing out of the hole in the artery, is given time to clot and form a firm plug. This normally takes five to seven minutes; but to be on the safe side it is best to maintain the pressure for at least ten minutes. Do not release the pressure after a few minutes to see if the bleeding has stopped, because if it has not stopped pressure will have to be applied again for a further ten minutes. If bleeding is severe it may be necessary to maintain pressure for fifteen minutes. This is an extremely long time under stressful conditions. Do not guess the time; watch a clock or ask someone to time you. It is best to use some form of dressing to apply the pressure but if one is not immediately available then anything will do – a handkerchief, a towel or even your shirt.

When the time has elapsed do not remove the dressing used to apply the pressure, because removing it may interfere with the clot which has formed. You should apply a firm bandage over this dressing (see illustrations on page 69) and start to plan the patient's transfer to hospital (see Chapters 5 and 6).

Control of bleeding from veins

When the oxygen and nutrients have been delivered to the cells by the arterial blood and the waste products and carbon dioxide have been

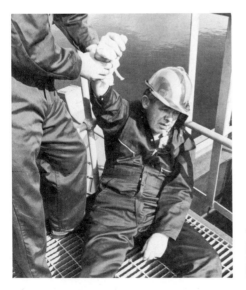

To stop severe bleeding raise the limb above the heart and apply direct pressure to the wound for ten to fifteen minutes.

removed from them, the blood becomes a bluish colour. It also flows more slowly because most of the energy of the heart has been spent in forcing the blood along the arteries and then through the tiny capillary channels in the body's organs. The blood then collects in the veins and is transported in these vessels back to the heart. The pressure in the veins is therefore much lower than that in the arteries.

When a vein is severed, the blood flows smoothly from it, and is bluish in colour. Venous bleeding, though, can still be a major problem. But it can easily be stopped in an arm or leg by laying the casualty on his back and raising the limb above the level of the heart and applying pressure to the wound.

The common site for pure venous bleeding is varicose veins in the leg. These tend to be very thin-walled and are therefore vulnerable. In any large wound there will be some venous bleeding because both veins and arteries are likely to be damaged. It is therefore important when dealing with any major wound to raise the part which is bleeding above the level of the heart, if this is possible. This will immediately reduce the venous bleeding and will slow by gravity the flow rate of the arterial bleeding. Applying pressure to the wound, as previously described, will then stop the arterial bleeding.

Bleeding from a limb
The casualty should be encouraged to sit or lie down. The limb should then be raised at the same time as pressure is applied. This allows gravity to be used to reduce the pressure.

When to use tourniquets
The best method of controlling bleeding is to raise the injury and apply pressure, as previously described above. Applying a tourniquet correctly stops the spurting arterial bleeding but may not stop the smoother venous bleeding. And tourniquets sometimes cause considerable damage to tissues. Their main danger is that they are sometimes forgotten. If they are left in place for too long (1½–2 hours) they starve the tissues beyond the band of oxygen causing them to die.

The two situations in which they may be used as a temporary time-saving measure for severely bleeding leg or arm wounds are:

1. In dealing with multiple casualties, when it would not be possible to spend fifteen to twenty minutes with one casualty in order to stop bleeding by direct pressure.
2. In a single casualty who either has more than one severely bleeding wound or is not breathing and thus requires immediate resuscitation.

A tourniquet is a constricting band made from a tie or a belt or some similar item which can be applied tightly enough above an arm or leg wound to stop the spurting arterial bleeding. A tourniquet must always be removed as soon as possible, and no later than twenty minutes after it was applied. If bleeding persists, then apply direct pressure to the wound as previously described.

We explain how to control different types of bleeding that may not be life-threatening in Chapter 4.

Unconsciousness

The unconscious casualty is the most vulnerable and can very easily die if he vomits and breathes the fluid into his lungs, or if his airway becomes blocked. The first thing to do when assessing a casualty is to determine whether he is conscious or unconscious.

The unconscious casualty

Treating the unconscious casualty is more important than finding out why he is unconscious. If he is not breathing or his heart is not beating the ABC of basic life support must be undertaken immediately, as described previously. When you have established that his airway is clear, he is breathing and his heart is beating, any bleeding should be stopped and any fractures immobilized (see Chapter 4). The casualty should then be placed in the recovery position (see below). When in this position, he is relatively safe from the effects of vomiting or of obstructing his airway with his tongue. He should not be left alone, though, and the first aider should remain with him until help arrives.

Recovery position

The recovery position is used for unconscious casualties who are breathing and whose hearts are beating. In our experience, we have found this procedure to be essential even for a casualty with a suspected spinal injury. Provided it is carried out slowly and carefully, taking every precaution to twist the back as little as possible, it can be very helpful. This is easier to do with more than one helper.

The illustrations overleaf show how to place someone in the recovery position. When in the recovery position the casualty lies with: .

1. His upper arm bent at the elbow and at right angles to the body
2. His upper leg bent at the knee and at right angles to support the lower body
3. His lower arm stretched out parallel with his body
4. His lower leg slightly bent at the knee

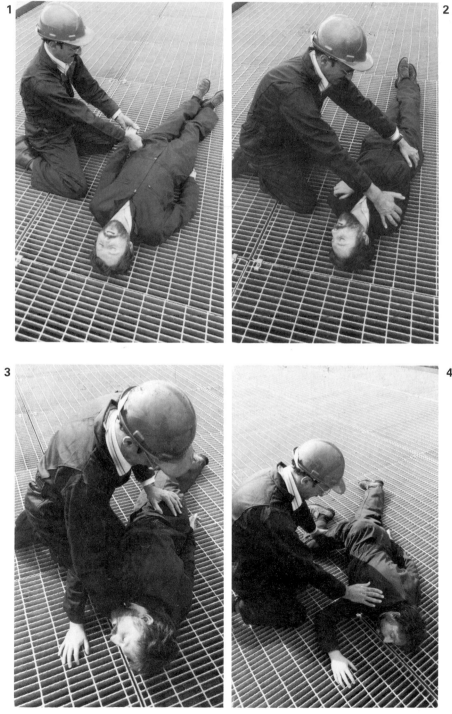

5. His head slightly turned to one side so that if he vomits he will not breathe in the vomit.

Continuing unconsciousness

The most common cause of unconsciousness offshore is head injury. It is important to be able to determine the level of consciousness of any unconscious casualty, particularly if you are asking for advice on further management or evacuation. It is best not to use words such as stupor and coma because these terms mean different things to different people. It is much better to use your own language to describe the casualty. A suggested classification of levels of consciousness is given below.

Levels of consciousness

Level 1   Full consciousness. The casualty is alert and able to answer questions normally.

Level 2   The casualty is drowsy. He is, however, easily roused (e.g. gives correct answer to simple questions) but relapses into a drowsy state.

Level 3   The casualty is unconscious. He can be aroused only with difficulty. He is aware of pain such as nipping of the skin but not of other external stimuli, such as being spoken to.

Level 4   The casualty is so deeply unconscious that he cannot be aroused at all.

Continuing care

Never give anything by mouth to an unconscious person, neither leave him alone. Place him in the recovery position and wait for help. If he has to be transported ashore and a diagnosis has not been made,

Recovery position technique (*opposite*)
1. Kneel down at the side of the casualty. To turn the casualty towards you, tuck the nearside arm under the body.

2. Before turning, cross the casualty's legs and lay the far-side arm over the chest. Turn the head towards you to prevent stress on the neck.

3. As you turn the casualty towards you, use your knees as a break to prevent the casualty turning over too quickly once he has reached the point of balance. Guide the head with your hand, keeping the mouth clear of the ground.

4. Pull the top knee and arm forward to stabilize the body. The casualty's airway is now safe, should vomiting occur.

remember that whatever is causing the unconsciousness may result in his breathing or heart stopping. The person escorting him ashore must therefore be in a position to detect this as soon as it occurs and take appropriate action.

Specific conditions associated with unconsciousness

Fainting

Fainting follows a temporary failure of the supply of oxygen to the brain. It may follow an emotional disturbance, but often occurs after sitting or standing in a hot stuffy atmosphere for a long period of time, which causes the blood available for carrying oxygen to pool in the legs.

There is usually a feeling of dizziness preceding loss of consciousness and the casualty becomes pale and sweaty. The pulse is usually slow – less than sixty beats per minute. This slow pulse rate, combined with rapid recovery of consciousness once the casualty is laid down, distinguishes fainting from the conditions associated with shock. In cases of shock the pulse is weak and fast and the casualty shows no signs of recovery (see next chapter).

If the patient feels faint, sit him down with his head between his knees. Loosen the clothing round his neck and waist and tell him to tighten the muscles in his legs to improve the blood circulation. If the casualty faints put him in the recovery position (see previously in this chapter). He should regain consciousness fairly quickly. If he does not, then send for medical help and continue to monitor his breathing and pulse.

Management after fainting   Following a faint there will be a period of instability of the circulation which will last for several hours. It is important that a casualty who has fainted should be kept lying down for some time after the event or he will faint again.

Epilepsy

Epileptic fits have occurred offshore and they are a particularly dangerous hazard. Despite rigorous screening procedures epilepsy can still occur because it can develop from alcohol or drug withdrawal, or head injury. It can also occur for the first time in an offshore worker at any age.

An epileptic fit is caused by an abnormal discharge of electrical energy inside the brain. A fit begins when the sufferer suddenly loses consciousness and falls to the ground writhing and twitching. Some epileptics may remain rigid for a few seconds and then start having convulsions. The casualty will breathe noisily and froth may come from his mouth. He may also be incontinent. Finally, his muscles will relax and he will regain consciousness. He will have lost his memory of recent events and will be confused.

What to do   Keep calm – watching an epileptic fit can be frightening; and adopt the following procedure:

1. Prevent him from banging his head on the ground. Try to protect his head by cushioning it but do not restrain it. Wipe the froth from his mouth. Do not become too worried about his breathing. Although he may become blue, he will spontaneously begin to breathe again.
2. Move objects out of the casualty's way so he does not hurt himself. Do not restrain his limbs but guide their movements and slow them down so that he does not injure himself.
3. It is commonly believed that something should be placed between the teeth of an epileptic to prevent him biting his tongue. Epileptics rarely, if ever, bite their tongues and attempts to place things between their teeth are likely to do more harm than good.
4. When the casualty recovers, make him rest and do not leave him until you are sure he is fully aware of his surroundings.
5. There is no place for an epileptic on an offshore installation, even though his condition may be controlled by drugs. Therefore, make sure that someone in authority knows that you have dealt with this situation.
6. Because an epileptic fit in a helicopter is potentially dangerous to all concerned, medical advice must always be sought before transporting anyone who has had an epileptic fit.

Emergency action summary

If you understand the basic functions of the body, what goes wrong when certain types of illness or injury occur and the reasons for the advice normally given to cope with certain situations, then you will be in a strong position to deal with emergency situations when they arise. If you merely learn lists of things to do without understanding why you should do them then you will probably forget them when an emergency arises. Also, if you come across a situation which has not been catered for in the list you will not know what to do.

A certain amount of panic is unavoidable when you first deal with

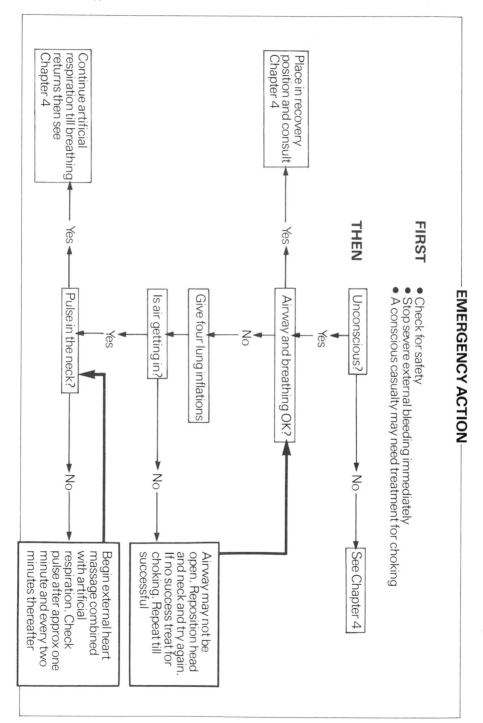

EMERGENCY ACTION

FIRST

- Check for safety
- Stop severe external bleeding immediately
- A conscious casualty may need treatment for choking

THEN

Unconscious? — No — See Chapter 4

Yes

Airway and breathing OK?

No — Give four lung inflations — Is air getting in?

Yes — Place in recovery position and consult Chapter 4

No — Pulse in the neck?

Yes — Continue artificial respiration till breathing returns then see Chapter 4

No — Begin external heart massage combined with artificial respiration. Check pulse after approx one minute and every two minutes thereafter

Airway may not be open. Reposition head and neck and try again. If no success treat for choking. Repeat till successful

a serious injury and it *is* therefore useful to have a basic list of priority measures which must be taken immediately if the casualty's life is to be preserved. To recap on what we have said in this chapter, ensure that:

1. The environment is safe for you (e.g. the casualty is not connected to an electric power socket or lying in a toxic atmosphere)
2. You know whether the casualty is conscious or unconscious (see page 47)
3. His airway is clear (see pages 30–2)
4. The casualty is breathing (see pages 30 and 33)
5. The heart is beating (see pages 30, 34 and 37)
6. Any bleeding has been stopped (see pages 42–5)
7. All fractures have been detected and immobilized (see Chapter 4)
8. If unconscious, put casualty in recovery position (see pages 45–7).

In this chapter we have dealt primarily with the emergency life-saving techniques that are the first priority in basic life support. In the next chapter we describe the next stage of action: the first aid that should be given for different types of injury and accident, once the casualty's immediate survival has been assured.

Opposite: Action flow chart for handling an emergency.

4. FIRST AID OFFSHORE

Assessing injury and illness

When the basic life-saving techniques, described in the previous chapter, have been given to the casualty, it is important to find out what is wrong with him. Begin by taking an accurate statement of what happened from the casualty himself or any onlookers. This is known as the history. For example, in the case of a fall from a height try to find out how far the man fell and what part of his body he landed on. If he landed on his feet, there may be fractures of the ankles and a fracture of the upper portion of the spine (see 'Indirect Fractures' on page 74). It would therefore be most important to examine the casualty's back and neck.

Recording the facts

The facts about an illness or accident should be written down and linked to the time they occurred (see charts page 202). The onset of illness is usually gradual but an accurate history is also required. Experience shows that memory is not an adequate substitute for written records. The first aider's notes should include:

- Pulse rate (see pages 55–6)
- Temperature (see below)
- Respiration rate (how many breaths are taken per minute).

The blood pressure should also be noted if it has been measured. All these should be recorded every thirty minutes, or as advised by the doctor onshore.

The casualty should be examined gently and any colour changes should be noted such as white skin due to shock, or blue skin caused by impaired circulation, or a blocked artery or vein. A rough idea of the casualty's temperature can be obtained by touching the skin under an area of clothing.

If one part of his body is painful, a hand should be passed gently over the skin to feel the consistency of the underlying bones and organs and to determine whether touch and a little gentle pressure makes the pain worse.

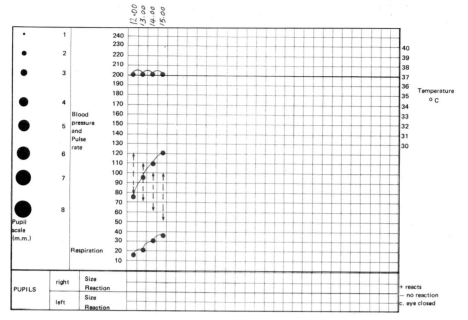

A reduced-size example of a chart used to record the measurements made when monitoring a seriously ill casualty. We have included full-size blank charts at the back of this book to use in an emergency. But if an appropriate chart is not available, use a piece of graph paper or draw your own.

The patient should be monitored continuously and any changes in his symptoms noted with the time they changed.

Passing on information
If the patient has to be evacuated and sent to hospital these records should accompany him as they are of great value to the hospital team. Whatever treatment you give the casualty it is important that the next man down the line should know what action you have taken. The badly injured casualty is more likely to survive if there is a smooth progression between the three phases of his management from immediate care, during transportation, to treatment in hospital.

Asking for help
When seeking advice from a doctor onshore you should provide him with all the relevant details of the injury. Five minutes spent assembling the facts in the correct order is time well spent and much more useful to the casualty than a garbled, panic-stricken call for help. A useful check-list when asking for help includes:

1. **The time** when the injury occurred or the illness began.
2. **The symptoms** in the order they occurred and at what time each appeared.
3. **The observations** made during the examination and the way in which they changed during monitoring.
4. **The recordings** of temperature, pulse rate and breathing rate, with the times of the measurements.
5. **A personal assessment** of the urgency of the situation and the degree of concern which the offshore attendant feels. This is particularly valuable if there is already some rapport between the offshore attendant and the doctor who is supporting him.

A clear message should allow the doctor to decide on the management of the patient, and whether back-up services or evacuation are required.

Continuing assessment

There may be a considerable delay before the casualty can be evacuated, for many reasons, such as the distance from the hospital or extreme weather conditions. In these cases it is necessary to be able, in a scientific way, to determine whether the patient is remaining stable, getting better or deteriorating. This information is also important when determining the urgency of obtaining help or undertaking evacuations in hazardous conditions. Assessing the clinical state of a casualty requires an understanding of the condition of shock. The presence or absence of shock and its rate of development provides the medical information required to determine the casualty's clinical state.

Shock

Shock was first described in 1896 by the American physician John Collins Warren, who termed it: 'a momentary pause in the act of death.' This is still the best description of shock, as it indicates precisely what is occurring. When shock is diagnosed the casualty has begun the process of dying and the situation is therefore urgent. Treatment of shock is designed to stop the process or at least to slow down its development.

Shock indicates that there is a failure in the supply of oxygen to the body's tissue cells. The supply of oxygen has been so reduced that the cells no longer function properly and will eventually die. The signs of shock are exactly the same, whatever the cause of the failure of the oxygen supply. There are three main causes:

1. Oxygen is not being delivered to the blood at the lungs. This may be caused by:
   - Breathing an atmosphere deficient in oxygen
   - Choking
   - A problem with the lungs (e.g. drowning or gassing)
   - A problem with the mechanics of the lung (e.g. crushed chest).

2. If the oxygen has passed into the blood at the lungs it may not be transported in sufficient quantities to the cells because there is not enough blood to carry it. Although the lungs breathe faster and the heart beats faster to overcome this deficiency they cannot compensate for a large blood loss. The reason for the shortage of blood may be obvious or obscure:
   - External bleeding
   - Internal bleeding (e.g. following crush injuries or fractures)
   - Loss of the fluid part of the blood (e.g. following damage to the skin, burns, or vomiting and diarrhoea in food poisoning)
   - Excessive sweating following injury in a hot climate

3. If oxygen enters the bloodstream through the lungs and there is sufficient blood to carry it to the cells, it still may not reach the cells in sufficient quantities if the pumping action of the heart is inadequate.

How to recognize shock

The skin is cold, pale and sweaty. This is because the body automatically directs the available blood to the brain, heart and kidneys, which are most vulnerable to oxygen deprivation. Sweat on the brow in association with cold, white skin are very distinctive characteristics of shock.

The breathing rate increases in an attempt to obtain more oxygen. The casualty's breathing becomes noisy, the movements becoming exaggerated.

The pulse rate rises progressively. You can only determine whether this is happening by counting the pulse rate at 15- or 30-minute intervals. The normal resting pulse rate is 60–90 beats per minute.

The pulse rate can be measured at the wrist (radial pulse) or the neck (carotid pulse). The radial pulse is measured at the front of the wrist about ½ in (1 cm) in from the thumb side (see illustration overleaf).

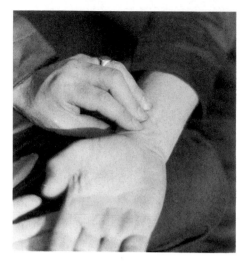

To feel the radial pulse, position your fingers on the thumb side of the wrist.

The carotid pulse is measured in the throat to one side of the windpipe (see illustration on page 37).

Feel the pulse with the second and third fingers of the hand. Count the number of beats in thirty seconds and multiply the number by two to give the rate per minute. Use a watch with a separate second-hand to time the pulse rate; do not estimate the time.

The surest way to determine shock is to count and chart the pulse rate. This is part of the standard monitoring process. The rate of rise or fall of the pulse rate is a good indication of the development or recession of shock and is important information to communicate to the doctor.

Blood pressure If you have been trained to measure blood pressure, monitor it. In shock the blood pressure will fall as the pulse rate rises. When the systolic pressure is less than the pulse rate the casualty's condition is usually grave.

Fear The patient will be afraid and anxious, though he may not know why and will need reassurance (see page 58).

Management of shock
It may be possible for the first aider to do a great deal in the management of shock, such as arresting bleeding, treating choking, treating drowning, removing the casualty from a toxic atmosphere, or giving artificial respiration or heart compression. Alternatively there may be little he can do in cases of internal bleeding or heart attack. However, there are certain non-specific actions which can be taken in all cases.

1. Reassure the casualty, talk to him, touch him and appear confident even though you may not feel it. This is extremely important because the state of shock will develop more rapidly if the casualty is anxious (see later in this chapter).
2. Lie the casualty down. This assists gravity to deliver whatever oxygen is available to the vital centres of the brain, heart and kidneys. Raising the legs may help, as it moves blood by gravity from the legs, which are less vulnerable to the effects of lack of oxygen to the vital centres.
3. If it is necessary to move the casualty do so slowly and handle him gently in case he has an unstable injury (e.g. broken bone) or you make internal bleeding worse by dislodging forming blood clots.
4. Depending on the circumstances, wet the casualty's lips if he is thirsty but do not give him a drink (see further discussion on fluids below).
5. Do not give alcohol to the casualty, it may make him feel better but can accelerate the development of shock.
6. Try to keep his temperature normal by keeping him warm in the cold or cool in the heat.
7. Keep a chart where the pulse rate, body temperature, breathing rate and any changes in the casualty's general state are noted against time (see page 53). These facts, as we have said, are vital for the medical officer ashore.

When to give fluids to drink

As a general rule casualties should be given nothing to drink if they are in shock or have sustained a serious accident. The reason for this is that they normally require an operation and fluid in the stomach may make this dangerous if they are to be given an anaesthetic. But in offshore medicine, there are some situations in which fluids can be given. It is important to assess each case and take appropriate action in different circumstances. This is why it is important to understand the basic theory of the various rules which are made for guidance in immediate care.

Burns
In casualties with burns, the likely cause of death in the early period after the burn is loss of fluid. The burnt casualty is not likely to require an operation immediately and since it may be many hours before he reaches hospital, it is advisable to start giving fluids right away even if he is badly injured or in early shock (see also pages 86–91).

A long time to wait
If it is going to take several hours to evacuate a badly injured casualty then it seems reasonable, on humanitarian grounds, that he should be given something to drink. Give him small quantities of bland fluids, such as water. Write down how much fluid the casualty has taken and when, and be sure that the receiving doctor is given the message.

Heat
In hot climates, if the casualty has been lying in the sun for several hours before help arrives it may be essential to give him fluids to drink before he is transported. He may be dying because of dehydration rather than his injuries.

Giving reassurance

Reassurance is very important for the injured person. If he is in pain, or fears for his life, he will be more likely to develop shock (see pages 54–7) than if he is comfortable and has confidence in the person helping him. Confidence must be instilled into the casualty, together with a strong feeling of reassurance. This is often difficult if an hour or two has to be spent with a seriously injured man before help arrives. Explain to him in a simple way the type of injury he has, how you have treated him and what further treatment he might need. Then talk to him about general topics such as the work he was doing before the accident. Do not keep asking him how he feels. This is annoying and will only make the casualty feel nervous.

Giving oxygen

A casualty in shock is suffering from a lack of oxygen to his body cells. Administering oxygen may help to maintain this vital supply. Oxygen may also be given to casualties with breathing difficulties caused either by a chest injury (see pages 72–3) or by gassing (see Chapter 8).

Equipment to administer oxygen is held on most offshore installations, normally in the sick bay. The cylinder has a valve which is opened by the key provided. The mask is then applied to the casualty's face. Many of these devices automatically provide sufficient oxygen to meet the casualty's needs by means of a demand valve. But if there is a flow meter, the best flow rate to use is 15–20 l/min.

Casualties who are developing shock often resist attempts to apply a mask onto the face. They may prefer the mask to be held an inch or two away from the face. This way they will still breathe enough oxygen, provided the flow rate is 15–20 l/min.

How to cope with pain

Information about a casualty's level of pain is important in diagnosing and assessing the severity of an injury, and serious problems have been caused when it was relieved before the hospital doctor had made his assessment. Nevertheless, continuing pain makes shock develop more quickly and in long journeys relief of pain is important. Where possible, discuss pain relief with a doctor before giving it.

Giving pain-relieving drugs
If you are advised by the onshore doctor to administer powerful analgesic drugs to a casualty, the doctor's instructions on dosage must be followed to the letter. The technique for injecting such a drug is illustrated below; and the following points should always be considered before the decision is taken to give strong painkillers, whether by injection or by mouth.

1. Powerful pain-relieving drugs usually depress the centre in the brain which controls breathing. They are thus especially dangerous in:
   - Head injury
   - Chest injury

When injecting an analgesic, pinch the skin at the top of the arm and insert the needle at approximately 45°.

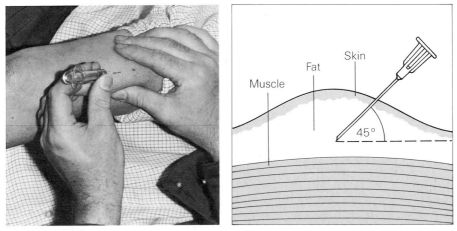

2. Administration of a powerful pain-relieving drug either by mouth or by injection may have no effect if the casualty's circulation is reduced by shock. If there is no effect do not repeat the dose, since it will all be absorbed when the shock passes off and the circulation improves. Under these circumstances, the casualty may stop breathing at that time.
3. A big man in a lot of pain will need a bigger dose of the drug to relieve the pain than a small man with only moderate pain.
4. An unconscious man with serious injuries is in no pain. He therefore does not need pain relief.

Gas-and-air analgesia

One of the safest methods of first-aid pain relief is by the use of Entonox, which is a 50 per cent mixture of nitrous oxide and oxygen. Entonox is effective and safe provided the casualty administers it himself. It is suitable for the majority of cooperative casualties in pain, and helps to alleviate the discomfort of changing dressings, the relocation of dislocated joints, and so on. One of the major advantages of using Entonox is that it does not mask the signs and symptoms of the injury when the casualty finally arrives in hospital. It is probably the best means of pain relief for a long journey if the equipment is available.

Entonox must not be used:

- For uncooperative or unconscious casualties who will be unfit to self-administer
- For casualties who have been exposed to pressurization (usually divers)
- In the presence of a naked flame, since the mixture supports combustion.

Storage and preparation of Entonox   When the gases are released from the cylinder they should form a constant composition mixture, but if the cylinder is cooled to below 18°F (−8°C) the contents separate out into liquid nitrous oxide and gaseous oxygen. If the gas is now released from the cylinder the initial delivery of gas will have a high oxygen content and eventually pure nitrous oxide will be delivered. To avoid this, the cylinder should be stored horizontally; it must not be stored in the open; and before use it must be at room temperature – above 50°F (10°C). If the cylinder has been exposed to a low temperature before use, the gases may have become separated, so the cylinder must first be warmed (*not* over a naked flame!) and then inverted at least three times in order to re-establish a stable mixture safe for pain relief.

How to administer Entonox   Entonox equipment is normally stored in the sick bay on offshore installations. The complete Entonox apparatus consists of the gas cylinder, a breathing valve similar to a diving demand valve which allows pressurized gas to be supplied at atmospheric pressure to the casualty when he breathes in, and a length of corrugated tubing connecting the cylinder and breathing valve to an anaesthetic face mask and expiratory valve. If the cylinder and breathing valve are stored separately they must be connected up according to the instructions on the apparatus.

Once the apparatus is ready to use, the casualty should be shown how to administer the Entonox to himself by holding the mask touching his face. Relief of pain comes on after a few breaths and may last several minutes. Once the analgesia takes effect the casualty should remove the mask. Continual breathing of the gas will lead to a very lightheaded feeling and sleepiness, and the mask should fall away. After several minutes of breathing air again the casualty will return to normal.

It is quite safe to take several breaths of the gas mixture repeatedly if required for pain relief, but regular breathing of Entonox over a long period of time (as in abuse of the gas) is dangerous.

Giving Entonox to a casualty   Allow the casualty to hold the mask over his nose and mouth and encourage him to breathe normally from the demand valve. He will remove the mask once the analgesia takes effect.

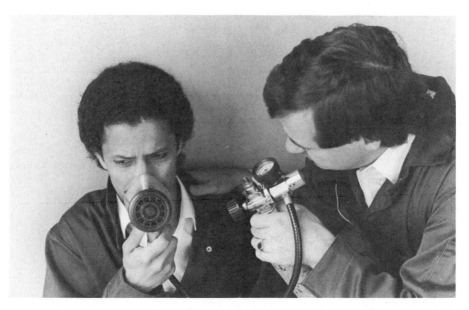

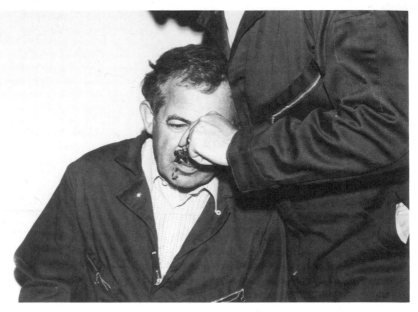

Stopping a nose bleed   Pinch the nose by the soft tissue just below the bony structure at the top of the nose. Ask the casualty to put his head forward and to breathe through his mouth.

Bleeding from specific areas

In the previous chapter we explained how to stop severe bleeding that was putting the casualty's life in immediate danger. Here we cover management of different types of bleeding that would need attention once the ABC of life support had been performed.

Nose bleeding
1. Apply pressure to the nose by pinching it between finger and thumb just below the bony structure at the top of the nose for at least ten minutes.
2. Hold the head forward to prevent the blood running into the windpipe.
3. The casualty should not sniff or blow his nose for several hours.

Bleeding from an ear
Following a blow on the head, bleeding from an ear suggests the skull may be fractured. Treatment is as follows:

1. No attempt should be made to stop this bleeding, because trapping it inside the skull may cause brain damage.

2. The casualty should be positioned so that the blood can flow out freely.
3. Put a clean pad over the ear to protect it from dirt.
4. Medical advice should be sought as soon as possible.

Control of bleeding in complicated wounds

Scalp In a head wound with an underlying fracture of the skull it may be difficult to apply direct pressure to the wound, as this may force the jagged ends of bone from a fractured skull into the brain. Because the scalp is liberally supplied with large blood vessels which do not readily constrict, it may bleed profusely. Indirect pressure should therefore be used around the wound by employing a ring pad (see illustrations below). In this way pressure can be applied well away from the wound until the bleeding has stopped.

Fractures A similar technique can be used for an open fracture (see page 75), where a piece of bone is protruding through the wound, or profuse bleeding makes it difficult or painful to apply direct pressure. In these cases a ring pad can be applied around the wound and indirect pressure used to stop the bleeding (see illustrations below).

A ring pad is made by twisting a triangular bandage or other material around its long axis and looping the ends together. It is placed round the protruding bone or the wound which may conceal a fracture. Pressure can then be applied on the pad to stop the bleeding. The pad also provides protection before splinting.

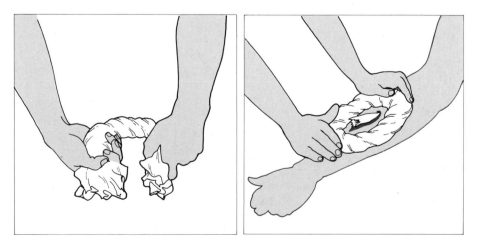

Special types of wounds

The following types of wound may all be encountered offshore:

Lacerated wound
The lacerated wound is the most common type suffered offshore. It is caused by a blow, such as that given by a hammer, which causes the tissue to burst open. Management involves stopping the bleeding (see pages 42–5 and 62–3), thoroughly cleaning the wound, and covering it with a pad and bandage designed to hold the wound edges together as closely as possible (see page 69). Then the casualty will need to be transported for specialist care.

Incised wound
An incised wound is made by a cutting tool or kitchen knife. It causes little tissue damage, but is dangerous because it allows foreign material to enter the body through the wound gap. The main aims of management are to prevent this contamination and to encourage the wound to heal with a firm scar. These are achieved by thorough cleaning of the wound (see pages 66–8) and then closing the edges together by means of dressing (see page 69). If a medically qualified person is available stitches may be used (see 67–8).

A lacerated wound caused by crushing.

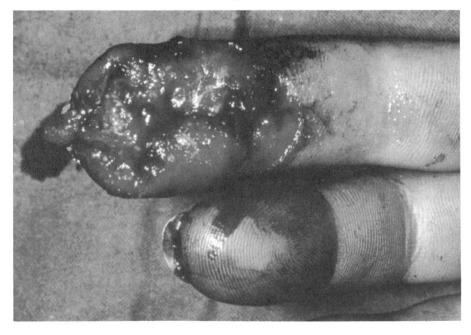

Abrasion

An abrasion results from a graze following a fall on a hard, rough surface. It appears to be a minor wound but it is probably one of the most painful because usually a large number of nerve endings are exposed and slightly damaged.

It is essential that this wound is thoroughly cleaned, although this may take some time if it is painful (see pages 66–8). If it is not thoroughly cleaned it will become infected, healing will be delayed and an ugly scar may result. Also, if oil is retained in the wound the skin may heal over it and leave a permanent tatooing type of blemish. The wound should be dressed with a sterile, non-adherent dressing and bandaged as shown on page 69.

Puncture wound

This wound is potentially the most dangerous of all because it often looks harmless. It may be caused by a sharp object such as a nail. Without exploring the wound it is impossible to know how far the object has penetrated the body or if it entered a body organ or joint space. Commonly, in this type of wound, fragments of clothing or dirt from the environment are driven into the body with the penetrating object. Because there is no clear opening to the surface it is this type

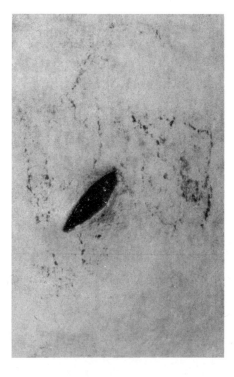

A puncture wound in the lower back. These wounds often look trivial but may penetrate very deep. In this example, the wound caused severe damage to one kidney.

of wound which is most commonly associated with the major infections of gas gangrene and tetanus. If bleeding is not severe and the casualty is showing no signs of shock, no special first aid care is necessary for the wound. Nevertheless, all puncture wounds must be seen by a doctor. The casualty should see the doctor urgently if the body trunk is punctured.

Amputation
Sometimes a whole limb is separated from the body when it is caught in moving machinery. In other cases part of a finger is partially or nearly removed. These injuries are more common in drillers than in other types of offshore workers and form a major portion of the injuries which need to be dealt with.

With modern techniques of microsurgery it is often possible to recon-nect a separated finger, toe or limb back onto the body. If such an injury occurs the separated portion of tissue should be transported with the patient in case some form of surgical reattachment can take place. If the tissue is merely placed in a bag with ice it will suffer cold injury and be damaged irreversibly. It is better to wrap it in a sterile dressing, place the wrapped tissue in a polythene bag and then to place the polythene bag in a refrigerated box or another polythene bag containing ice chippings. Rapid transport is essential under these circumstances as the tissue will only survive for approximately two hours before suffering irreversible changes due to lack of oxygen.

Wound care

If the casualty has had severe bleeding (see Chapter 3) it must, of course, be stopped as quickly as possible, but in this case wound cleaning should not be carried out offshore. Wound cleaning should only be performed offshore for minor wounds, such as cuts and grazes, where bleeding is not a problem.

If there is an object embedded in the wound, do not pull it out because it may be plugging a damaged artery or lying next to a nerve. If it is pulled out it may do further damage by severing the artery or nerve completely. To cover the period of time before the casualty receives medical attention dress the wound by placing a ring pad or several ring pads around it before adding a thick pad and bandage (see illustrations opposite).

Wound cleaning
1. If the wound is dirty, it should be washed in running water if possible.

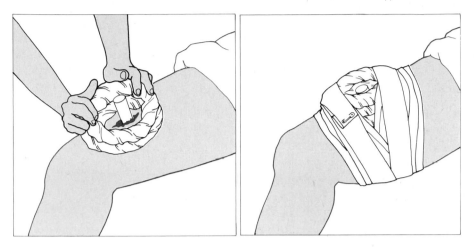

A series of ring pads can be used to build up protection around a protruding foreign body. These are then bandaged in place to prevent movement (of the object) in any direction.

2. Since it will usually be many hours before the casualty is seen by a doctor an antiseptic solution should be used in the water if possible. Instructions are usually given on the antiseptic bottle and it is important to use a solution of antiseptic in water rather than in spirit. If you have no antiseptic, clean the wound with soap and water.
3. Gently clean the area around the wound with the antiseptic solution using a succession of moist cloths. Each stroke should be from the wound edge away from the wound and you should begin from the middle of the wound and work outwards.
4. Dry the skin gently.
5. Put a dressing on the wound large enough to cover it and extend beyond it.
6. Bandage a thick pad over the dressing (see illustrations on page 69).
7. Tetanus is always a risk with contaminated wounds. It is advisable for those who work offshore to be actively immunized against tetanus. If in doubt about tetanus take medical advice.

Stitching
After thorough cleaning, a doctor or paramedic will often close a wound by stitches. But when the wound has been left open for a long time the possibility of contamination from the atmosphere is so great

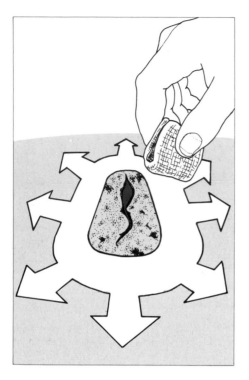

When cleaning a wound, use a new sterile swab, soaked in antiseptic, for each stroke. Each cleaning wipe should be directed outwards, away from the centre of the wound.

that there is a considerable chance of infection developing in the closed wound if it is stitched. This can happen offshore because there may be a considerable delay between sustaining an injury and delivering the casualty to a centre where stitching is feasible. If the wound has been open for more than six hours it is normally recommended that primary stitching should not take place until it can be determined that the wound has not been grossly infected.

Head injuries

Head injuries are fairly common offshore and are usually associated with the following:

- An object such as a tool being dropped from a height onto the head
- A swinging object striking the head, for example something on a crane hook or the crane hook itself

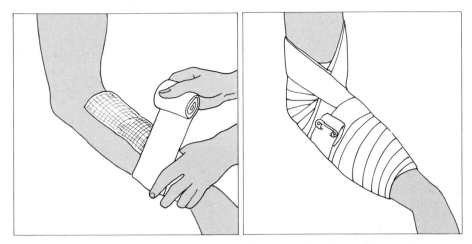

A bandage should be firm enough to hold the dressing in position and prevent further bleeding but not so tight as to limit the circulation. Make a figure of eight around a joint to prevent the bandage slipping and to provide protection for the joint without preventing movement.

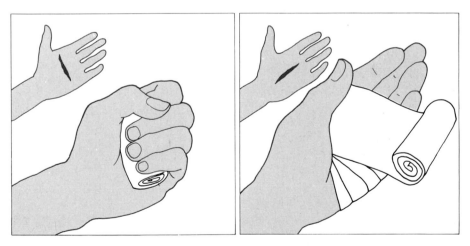

Always bandage a wound in a way which will hold the wound edges together. In a mainly crosswise wound of the hand a pad should be grasped and the fist bandaged to look like a boxing glove.

In a lengthwise wound of the hand it is best to apply a bandage from side to side so that the wound edges are held together. If the finger tips are unaffected they should be left outside the bandage so that circulation of blood to the hand can be checked.

- Falling down a ladder and striking the head on the steps or the rails
- Striking the head when balance is lost due to violent motion on a ship or a helicopter
- A helicopter pilot may strike his head on an object on the flight deck during an emergency.

All casualties who have received a blow to the head, particularly if unconsciousness followed, should have medical attention. They should also be observed for twenty-four hours in case further neurological problems develop. If casualties with head injuries have to be moved great care must be taken in case the skull or spine are fractured (see pages 74–85).

The main problem in head injury
The brain is a delicate organ which is encased in the bony skull for protection. The main problem with head injury is that if the brain is damaged or bleeding occurs inside the skull the blood will accumulate there and the brain may swell. Because the brain is enclosed in the rigid skull and cannot expand, when it swells or when blood accumulates it becomes damaged. This often happens when the skull is fractured. Pressure then increases inside the skull either from swelling of the brain following injury or from bleeding and it may be necessary for a doctor to relieve the pressure by surgical means.

Anyone who has had a blow to the head should be asked to report any unusual symptoms occuring during the following forty-eight hours. These include dizziness, a change in vision, drowsiness or headaches. If the casualty reports any unusual symptoms medical advice should be taken immediately.

Head injury and unconsciousness
An immediate cause for concern is a head injury associated with a period of unconsciousness. Because the brain may bleed or swell even after consciousness has been regained, a patient who has been unconscious is normally kept very quiet and observed closely for twenty-four hours after regaining consciousness. Ideally this observation should take place in hospital but if this is not possible the first aider should check for the following:

The level of consciousness should be monitored every fifteen minutes and noted according to the suggestions made on page 00. If the level of consciousness is becoming deeper this is a cause for concern.

It is not possible to distinguish unconsciousness from deep sleep, so the casualty must be awakened every fifteen minutes during the first twenty-four hours to determine his waking level of consciousness. This will do nothing for your popularity!

The pulse rate This should be measured at the same time and the reading noted (see pages 55–6). In all other situations where the patient is deteriorating and bleeding, the pulse rate tends to rise. In head injury, though, the pulse rate often tends to fall because of the pressure which may be being applied to the brain centre controlling heart rate.

The eyes should be observed at the same time. The anatomical components responsible for eye movements and vision have connections from the eyes to various parts of the brain. Any changes in eye response may indicate problems in localized parts of the brain. Some of these signs can only be observed if the patient is conscious but some can be observed even if he is deeply unconscious. The danger signs are:

- Unequal shape or size of pupils
- Pupil does not react when light is shone on it.

Bleeding within the skull as the result of a blow to the head can create pressure capable of disturbing the nerve supply to the eyes. This may result in unequal-sized pupils.

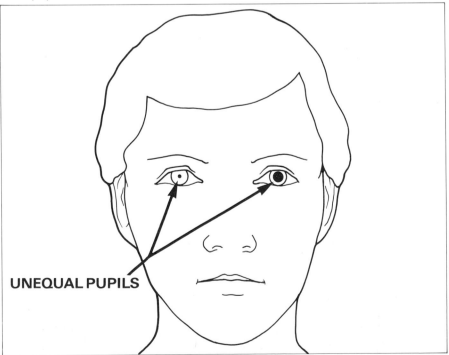

UNEQUAL PUPILS

These signs can be tested for in the same way the eye is examined for a foreign body (see page 91).

Danger signs
The danger signs are:

- Deepening levels of unconsciousness
- Slowing of pulse rate
- Any of the eye signs listed above.

If any of these things occur medical advice should be sought urgently and the casualty transported to a place where he can get surgical help. He may stop breathing at any time, and once breathing has ceased his heart may stop beating. The first aider escorting the casualty ashore must be aware of this and be competent at artificial respiration and heart compression in case they are necessary (see Chapter 3).

The most serious and urgent emergency situation occurs when a casualty who has been unconscious following a head injury regains consciousness and subsequently slides back into unconsciousness. This sign demands the most urgent action if the casualty's life is to be saved and he must have medical attention immediately.

Chest injuries

Chest injuries account for 5 per cent of offshore injuries and are often caused by crushing resulting from the movement of cargo in supply boats on high seas. Crushing causes multiple fracture of the ribs. The sharp ends of the ribs may also cause injury to the lungs. Whether this happens or not, the mechanics of breathing will be disturbed. The patient will become progressively short of oxygen and may die from lack of oxygen if the injury is severe. The patient should be carefully observed for the early signs of shock (see pages 55–6), which indicate that the supply of oxygen to the body cells is reduced.

What to do

1. Any wound on the chest wall should be immediately covered with a dressing (a handkerchief will do in an emergency) and sealed with an airtight material such as a polythene bag to prevent air passing in or out of the chest wall (see illustration opposite).
2. Breathing difficulties can be alleviated by sitting the casualty upright and leaning him towards his injured side. In this position his healthy lung has room to expand; the gut is also pushed

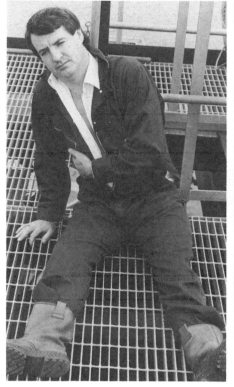

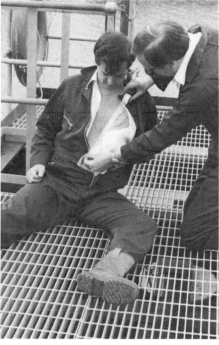

A casualty with a chest injury usually finds breathing easier if he is sitting up and leaning towards the injured side.

A dressing and plastic cover should be taped to an open chest wound. This will help to prevent air passing in and out of the chest.

downwards leaving more room for expansion of the lungs. But if you suspect the casualty has a back injury, for example after falling from a height, do not move him unless absolutely necessary.

3. Give oxygen if oxygen administration equipment is available (see pages 58–9).

4. Observe the casualty carefully for any signs of shock (see pages 55–6). If shock seems to be developing the casualty requires specialist help. Ideally he needs the attention of a qualified anaesthetist. This is probably provided most rapidly by bringing an anaesthetist with ventilation equipment to the offshore structure on the evacuating helicopter.

Broken bones

Bones provide support for the various tissues in the body and protect the brain, heart and lungs. They also act as levers in association with the muscles to allow movement to take place. If a bone is broken or damaged these functions may be lost so that movement of the limbs or digits takes place imperfectly or not at all. The shape of the bone may change and you may notice that the body's symmetry is disturbed. Broken ends of bones may penetrate the brain, heart or lungs causing serious damage.

Fractures at the point of impact

A fracture is a broken bone, normally caused by a direct force such as a kick or a blow. Bones may also be broken after a fall; a fall on an outstretched hand, for instance, may cause a fracture of the wrist. A fall from a height when the casualty lands on his feet usually results in a fracture of the ankle where the force of impact is concentrated.

Indirect fractures

Fractures are sometimes caused by indirect force, when the shock wave passes along a limb and fractures a bone at a distance from the point of impact. Thus, a fall on an outstretched hand may not result in a fracture of the wrist but in a fracture of the collar bone. Similarly a fall on the feet from a height may not cause a fracture of the ankle but a fracture of one of the delicate bones in the neck.

Fractures caused by indirect force are much less common than those caused by direct force. But they do occur and for this reason no casualty should be moved until he has been thoroughly examined and the possibility of indirect fractures, occuring away from the point of impact, excluded.

Fracture symptoms

Pain   A fracture is always associated with considerable pain, particularly when the injured part is moved.

Loss of function will be obvious in the injured part, for example the casualty will not be able to walk on a broken leg or write with a broken wrist.

Swelling and bruising are likely because of internal bleeding. There may be deformity but this may only be obvious when both limbs — both arms, for instance — are compared.

Shock   Major fractures can result in considerable internal bleeding. The soft tissues associated with the fracture may be extensively damaged by the sharp bone ends and may bleed profusely. Where this possibility is suspected the casualty should be observed carefully for the development of the signs of shock (see pages 55–6).

Types of fracture

Closed fracture   This is the most common type of fracture. The broken ends of bones are not associated with an overlying wound and they do not cause internal injury or protrude through the skin. This is the simplest type of fracture and it is important not to convert it to a more serious type by clumsy handling and management. In normal circumstances, with proper treatment this type of fracture heals readily with a minimum of residual damage.

Open fracture   The broken ends of the bone are exposed to the outside environment through an overlying wound. The ends of the bone may or may not protrude through the wound or the skin. This is a much more serious injury than the closed fracture because infection can easily develop in the exposed bone ends thus delaying and complicating the healing process. This type of injury often takes much longer to heal than a closed fracture and it may be associated with imperfect healing

Three different types of fracture: closed (left), open (centre) and complicated right.

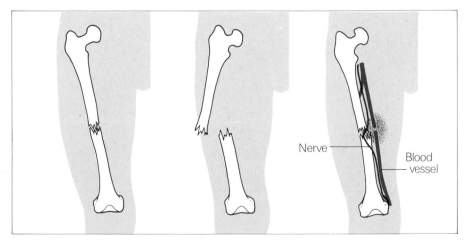

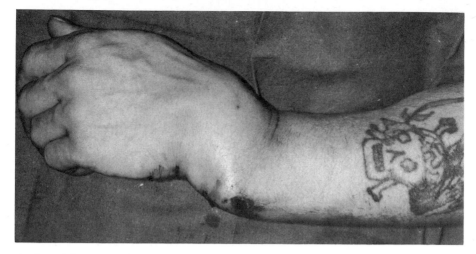

A closed fracture of the wrist.

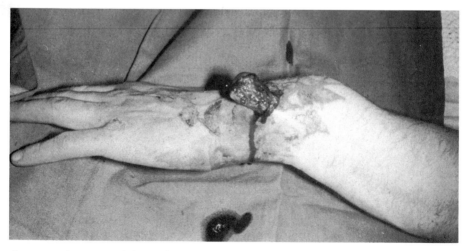

An open fracture of the wrist.

and permanent disability. It is therefore vital not to convert a closed fracture into an open fracture by mismanagement.

Complicated fracture   The ends of the broken bone causes internal damage to the body organs and/or the blood vessels. In a complicated limb fracture a nerve or a blood vessel is often caught between the bone ends. For this reason the sensation and blood supply to the hand

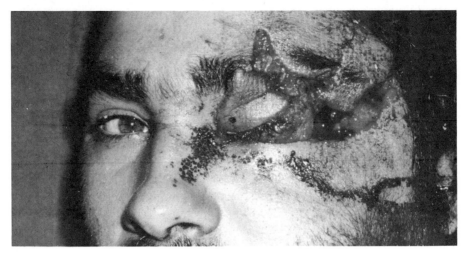

A complicated fracture. The fracture of the bone around the eye is complicated because it involves the eye itself.

or foot should be assessed following a fracture of the arm or leg before immobilization or further action is taken.

General treatment of fractures
1. Tell the casualty not to move. Do not move him unless his life or yours is in danger. Treat him where he is. If he must be moved, temporarily immobilize him (see below) before moving him as short a distance as possible.
2. Stop any bleeding and treat severe wounds (see pages 42–5 and 62–8). Cut away restrictive clothing and rings if possible. If these areas begin to swell, such restrictions will impair the circulation.
3. Support the injured area until the fracture has been immobilized to prevent further damage.
4. Immobilize the fractured area with bandages and splints if necessary (see below).
5. All fractures require medical attention.

Immobilization
This is carried out to prevent further damage to the fracture area. It can be done by bandaging one area of the body against another, or by bandaging a splint to the affected part.

In general do not move the injured part, for example if bandaging both legs together move the good leg towards the bad one.

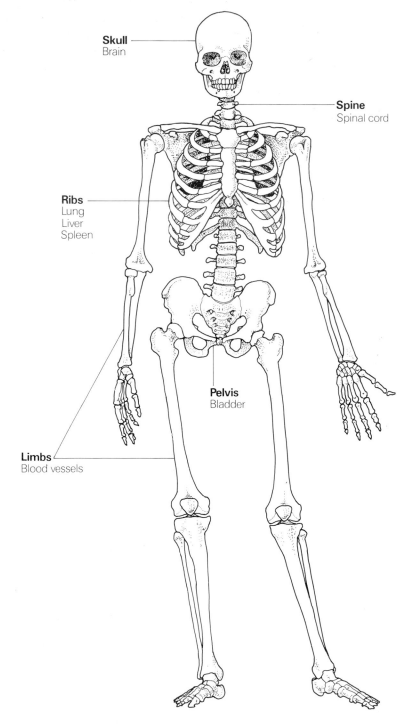

Skull
Brain

Spine
Spinal cord

Ribs
Lung
Liver
Spleen

Pelvis
Bladder

Limbs
Blood vessels

Immobilize the fracture area and the joints either side or end of it. To make the casualty more comfortable put thick padding between the two parts of the body which are bandaged together. Towels or socks can be used for padding. Belts, scarves and towels can be used instead of bandages, but make sure buckles on belts are covered so they do not hurt the casualty.

Bandages should be applied firmly but not tightly. They should not alter blood circulation or cause pain. Check them every fifteen minutes because the injury may swell causing the bandages to become too tight. Do not have a bandage directly over the suspected fracture area. Always tie knots on the uninjured side.

If splints are required they should be long enough to immobilize the joints either side of the fracture.

Air splints   These are inflated by mouth and are used for immobilizing limb fractures (see page 83).

Vacuum splints   The air is sucked out of a mass of expanded polystyrene pellets to form a solid mould around the injured area, without in any way altering the position of the limb. They are held in place by Velcro straps. Different types of vacuum splints are available for neck and limb fractures (see page 84).

Box splints   These are used mainly for fractures of the legs and arms. They are quick and easy to put on and are completely weatherproof (see page 84).

Spinal boards   These are pieces of wood which are useful for immobilizing neck and high spinal injuries. They are held in position by belts and buckles. These are now almost outdated by the Hines cervical splints, which are preferable.

Hines cervical splint   This is a moulded plastic collar and back piece which is used to immobilize the neck. It is held in place with Velcro straps (see page 85).

Improvized splints   If no splints are available, cardboard, folded newspaper, or pieces of wood covered with cloth to guard against splinters may be used.

Opposite: Complicated fractures of the skeleton will weaken the protective, structural function of the bone framework.

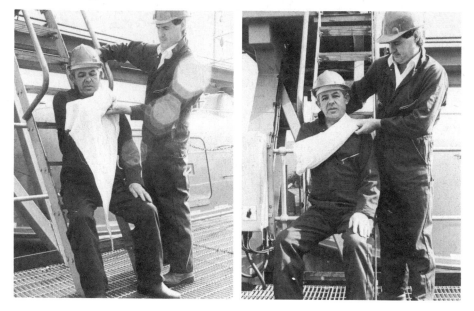

High sling (*above*)
1. This can be used to raise the hand if it is bleeding or swollen. Raise the injured arm across the body resting the hand on the opposite shoulder. Wrap the sling over the top of the arm and tuck it underneath to hold the arm firmly.

2. Bring the dangling end of the sling under the arm and round the back, and tie it securely to the other end of the sling at the side of the neck.

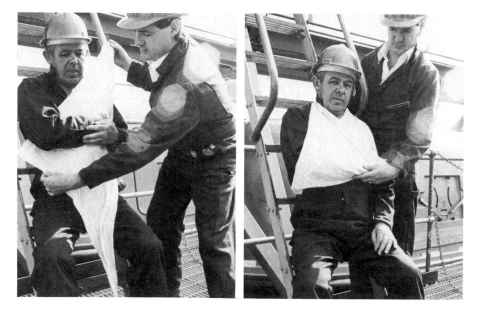

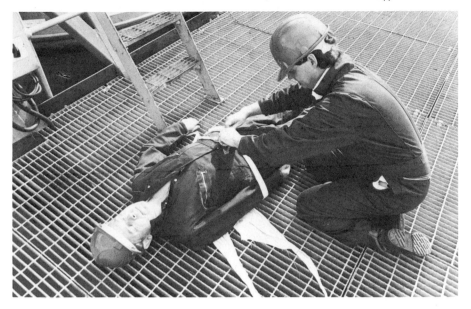

Arm immobilization using slings (*above & below*)

1. If you cannot bend the injured arm, strap the arm to the side of the body. First pass the slings under the casualty.

2. Tie the slings firmly along the length of the arm so it is fully supported. The knots should be secured away from the injured arm.

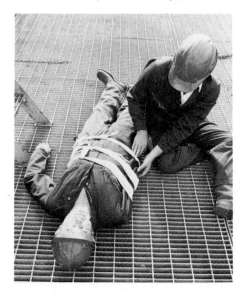

Horizontal sling (*opposite*)

1. This should be used for a fractured arm which can bend at the elbow. Lie the sling against the body and position the injured arm horizontally across it.

2. Fully support the weight of the arm in the sling and tie a secure knot at the side of the neck.

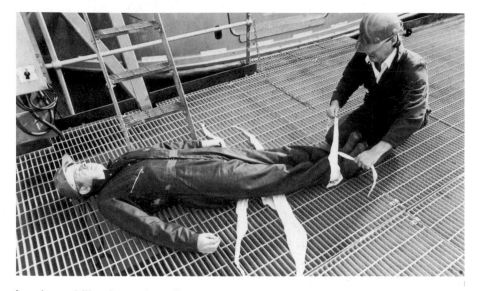

Leg immobilization using slings

1. Pass the slings gently under the casualty. First, secure the feet by tying a knot on the side of the boot.

2. Then tie the legs firmly together with the remaining slings, securing the knots on the uninjured side.

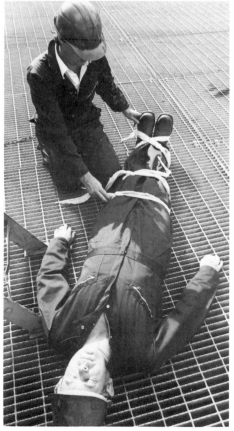

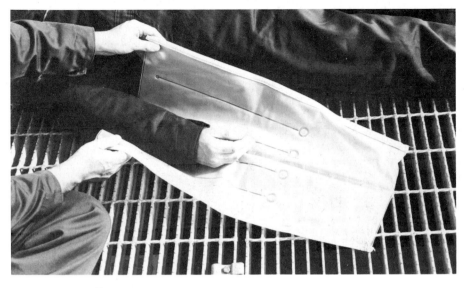

Applying air splint to the arm
1. Pass the air splint gently under the arm and fasten the zip.

2. Pull the nozzle out and inflate the splint by mouth until it feels firm and supportive. Be careful not to restrict blood flow.

3. Finally, check that the splint is clear of the fingertips so you can monitor circulation.

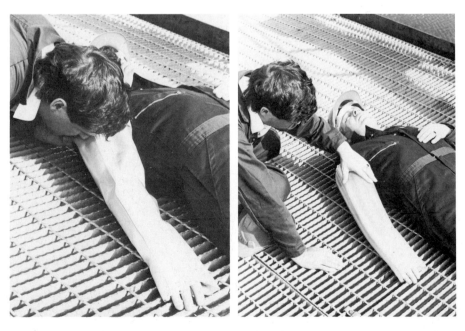

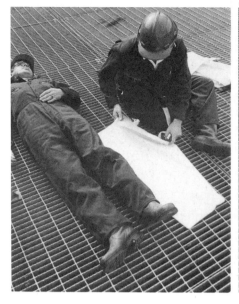

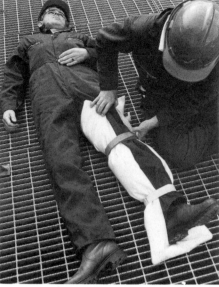

Applying vacuum splint to the leg
1. Gently pass the splint under the injured leg.

Box splint technique
1. Position the splint ready for use alongside the leg.

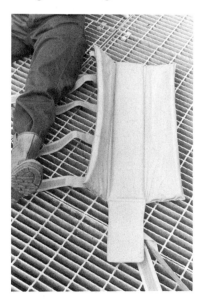

2. Hold the splint in position with Velcro straps. Suck the air out of the splint through the two-way valve at the nozzle. The vacuum created will provide a rigid cast to support the leg.

2. Gently slide the injured leg on top of the splint and attach it firmly with Velcro straps.

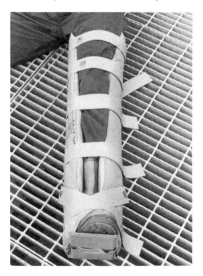

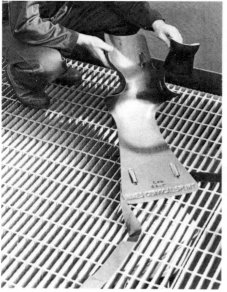
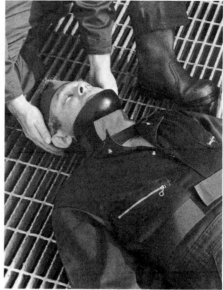

Hines cervical splint

1. This splint consists of a rigid collar and moulded back piece which is fastened to the body with Velcro straps.

2. Slide the back piece into position under the casualty and secure it by means of three Velcro straps around the forehead, neck and abdomen.

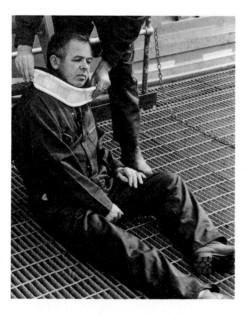

A Velcro collar can be used to support the neck when injury is suspected.

Burns

In any major accident offshore burns will be the greatest immediate first-aid problem. In normal circumstances most burns on an offshore structure are caused by welding torches or minor accidents in the living quarters. Burns damage the skin by the application of excessive heat to the surface of the body. The aim of treatment is to cool the burn as quickly as possible, because heat retained in the tissues can cause continuing damage to the body's cells.

The function of the skin is to prevent organisms from the environment getting into the body and to prevent the water content of the body from escaping. When the skin is damaged by burning the escape of water from the body may lead to shock (see page 54) and to death if the burn is severe. In those casualties who survive the loss of water, death may result from infection.

Broadly speaking there are two types of burns:

Superficial burns

These do not destroy all the skin cells, so the skin will eventually regenerate from those cells which are left undamaged. A superficial burn usually has a red surface and is painful because the nerve endings in the skin have been damaged but not destroyed.

This diagram shows the depth to which a burn can penetrate the skin, depending on the degree of burn: superficial, partial and full thickness.

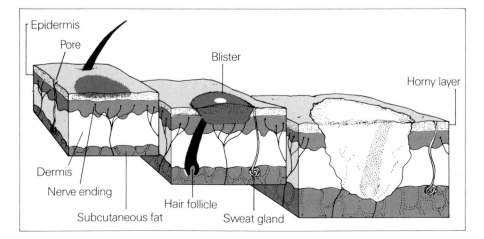

Deep burns

All the skin cells are irreversibly damaged in a deep burn and regeneration of the skin cannot therefore occur. The skin surface can only be replaced by skin grafting. A deep burn may not be painful because the nerve endings in the skin have been destroyed. It has a dirty grey colour.

Aims of treatment

The main aims of treatment for all types of burns are:

- To remove the source of heat
- To cool the skin area effectively
- To prevent infection
- To remove constrictions such as rings and boots before swelling of the affected tissue takes place.

Immediate action

1. If the casualty's clothes are on fire, put the fire out either by throwing water over the clothes or by smothering the casualty in a thick blanket, rug or jacket.
2. Remove the source of heat or move the patient away from it.
3. Immediately cool the burn with cold water (sea water can be used). Cooling is best done with running water. If this is not possible a large pad soaked in water can be put on the burned area and water continually poured over it. This process should be continued for at least ten minutes and until the pain is eased. The heat in the tissues may have built up rapidly but it will take at least ten minutes to ensure that the excess heat has all been removed.
4. Remove anything tight, such as rings, belts and boots straight away, as the burned area will begin to swell. Do not remove burnt clothing which has stuck to the skin; it will be sterile following the fire and trying to remove it may cause more damage to the few remaining skin cells. It is best therefore, to wrap the patient in clean dressings. If there are no dressings, a sheet or a pillow case can be used. Do not use fluffy materials as they will stick to the wound.
5. Do not apply any ointment to the burn at this stage.
6. Do not burst any blisters which may form. They provide protection against infection and keep vital body fluid in. In any case, the surface skin of the blister will fall off when healing has taken place below it.
7. The main cause of death in the early period following a severe burn is loss of fluid. This is one form of injury where the patient

should be encouraged to drink water from the beginning. It is unlikely that he will require a surgical operation on reaching hospital and fluid intake could save his life. If he is conscious, he should drink about half a cup of water every ten to fifteen minutes.

Special burns

Burns of the face   When the face is burned, even slightly, there is the possibility that hot gases or flames may have been inhaled, causing swelling of the linings of the breathing passages. Such a complication of burns is serious and often leads to death if there is a delay in evacuating the patient to intensive care facilities. During evacuation, watch for problems with the airway and breathing. Sips of cold water may help to reduce the swelling. If the casualty develops breathing difficulties you may have to give him oxygen (see pages 58–9).

Electrical burns normally cause a very localized burn. The main danger of a massive electric shock is stoppage of the heart. But the severity of

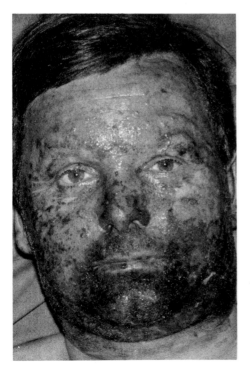

Facial burns. It is very important to check the airway is clear in a casualty with facial burns, as swelling due to heat may cause a fatal obstruction.

an electrical burn may be underestimated. Remember that the heat from the burn is often transmitted along nerves and blood vessels, so there may be excessive heat passing along under the skin. This can result in the appearance of much damaged tissue several days later if the whole limb is not cooled by immersion in running water for ten minutes.

Chemical burns are caused by strong acids or alkalis reacting with the skin to produce heat. These substances are found offshore in batteries, laboratories and in the chemicals used to modify crude oil. Treat as follows:

1. Flood the burned area with running water to dilute and remove the chemical. Make sure that the water drains away safely and not, for instance, into the boots!
2. Any contaminated clothing should be removed as rapidly as possible, but avoid contaminating yourself.
3. When the chemical has all been removed from the burn area and the pain has decreased, apply a clean dressing and treat in the same way as other burns.
4. For chemical burns to the eye see pages 92 and 94.

Priority of evacuation for burns victims
All burns covering an area larger than two whole fingers should be seen by a doctor. In a disaster offshore, where there are large numbers of casualties with burns, it may be necessary to decide an order of priority for evacuation. Since the immediate threat to life is loss of body fluid through the burned area of skin, the severity of a burn can be determined by the surface area of the damaged skin. The so-called 'rule of nines' is used for this (shown in the illustration overleaf), in which the upper limbs are said to represent 9 per cent of the surface of the body; the head and neck a further 9 per cent; the lower limbs 18 per cent each; the front and back of the torso 18 per cent each; and the genitalia 1 per cent.

Burns, though, do not cover such precise anatomical areas and it can be difficult, even with this rule, to determine the damaged surface area. Another way of calculating the area involved is based on the knowledge that the palm of the casualty's hand (excluding his fingers) represents 1 per cent of his body surface area. By using both these methods it is usually possible to determine with sufficient accuracy the surface area involved in a burn.

If the transportation facilities to hospital are limited, priority should always be given to the casualties with burns covering 30–60 per cent

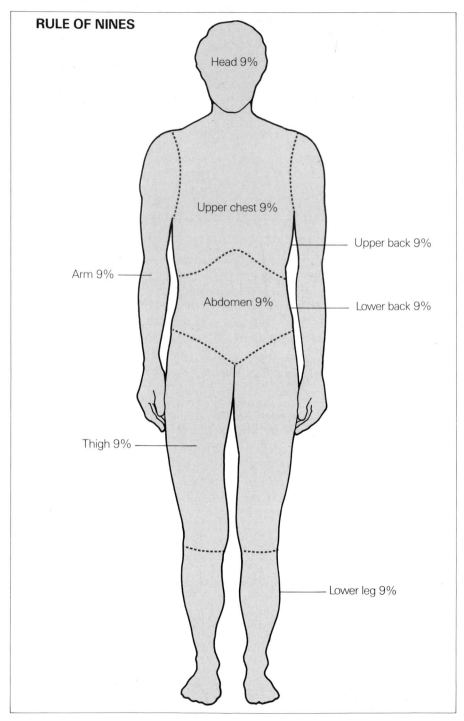

RULE OF NINES

Head 9%

Upper chest 9%

Upper back 9%

Arm 9%

Abdomen 9%

Lower back 9%

Thigh 9%

Lower leg 9%

of their body surface area. These patients are likely to die unless they receive medical attention urgently. If the surface area is greater than 60 per cent the casualty has little chance of survival even with medical aid. The second priority should be casualties with burns covering 9–30 per cent of their body area. Burns of less than 9 per cent take final priority because they can be managed adequately by first aid treatment for a limited period of time.

• Evacuate first:	30–60 per cent body area burns
• Then:	9–30 per cent body area burns
• Then:	Greater than 60 per cent body area burns
• Evacuate last:	Less than 9 per cent body area burns.

Eye injuries

Foreign bodies in the eye
This is a very common injury offshore, where there is a large amount of dust and where small fragments of metal often get into the eye, causing great pain and inflammation. We strongly recommend that workers offshore adhere strictly to their company's policy on wearing safety goggles, as this will prevent many unnecessary eye injuries.

If a worker does complain of a foreign body in his eye, the correct action to take is:

1. Tell the casualty not to rub his eye as this may embed the foreign body in the eye causing further damage.
2. Ensure he moves away from the environment where there are contaminating objects in the air.
3. Sit the casualty down facing the light and ask him to follow your finger with his eyes while keeping his head still. This allows you to examine his eye when it is rotated, first of all to the right, and then to the left. To determine if the foreign body is under the lower eyelid, ask the casualty to look upwards and pull the lower eyelid down.
4. To determine if the foreign body is under the upper eyelid ask the casualty to look down. Grasp the upper eyelashes and roll the eyelid up and over as shown in the illustration overleaf. This also allows you to examine the under surface of the eyelid where the foreign body may be embedded. Once found, the foreign body can be removed with the moistened corner of a clean handkerchief.

The rules of nines (*opposite*): Dividing body area up in this way helps the severity of burns to be assessed quickly.

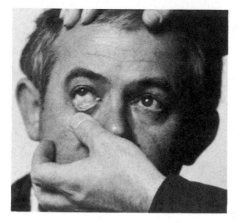
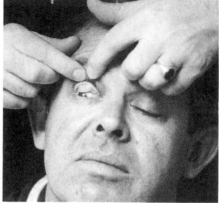

When looking for a foreign body under the lower eyelid, use the thumb to pull down the lid and ask the casualty to look upwards without moving his head. Use the corner of a handkerchief to remove the foreign body.

When looking for a foreign body under the upper eyelid, gently raise the eyelid by pulling the upper eyelashes upwards with thumb and index finger. Pull the eyelid back over the tip of your other index finger.

5. Do not attempt to move any object in the eye which is:
   - On the pupil or iris (the coloured part of the eye)
   - Embedded in the eye
   - Not visible. In this case close the eyelid, cover the eye with a soft pad held in place with a loose bandage and obtain medical help.

     Remember that the closed eye will still move in sympathy with the other eye. If it seems necessary to prevent eye movements then both eyes must be closed. If this is done, the patient must not be left alone until he reaches medical care because the total removal of vision can be a frightening experience.

The casualty must be seen by a medic or doctor in any of the three cases above.

Chemical contamination of the eye

This occurs most commonly in laboratory work offshore. The eye may be contaminated by corrosive chemicals such as acid splashes or drilling mud. Chemical contamination must be treated quickly if the vision is

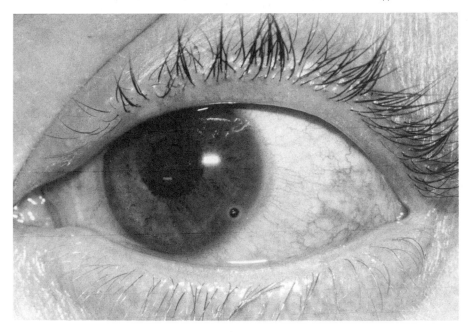

If the foreign body does not move around the cornea, as in this example, the first aider should not attempt to remove it.

Front view of the eye.

When covering an injured eye with a patch, tape it loosely to close and protect the eye.

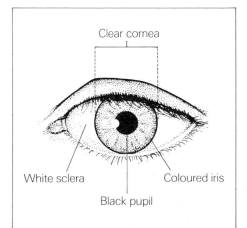

Clear cornea

White sclera

Coloured iris

Black pupil

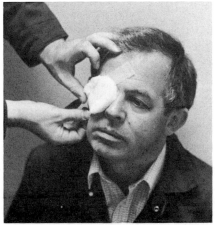

to be saved. The aim of treatment is to dilute and remove the chemical from the eye as quickly as possible.

1. Tilt the casualty's head towards the injured side and, holding a container filled with cool, fresh water close to the eye, pour the water into the eye from the nose side outwards to remove the chemical. Do not pour the water from a height, as this could cause discomfort. Continue this for at least ten to fifteen minutes. This may be difficult to achieve as the patient will be in severe pain but the longer the chemical is in contact with the delicate tissues of the eye the more likely it is that permanent damage will occur. Make sure that the other eye is not contaminated by the washing.
2. It is unnecessary to use neutralizing agents. Finding them may waste time and the urgent application of water is the treatment of choice.
3. After thorough washing, the eye should be covered with a dressing and the patient referred for immediate medical attention.

Arc eye

This occurs when a worker is temporarily blinded by looking at the bright light of a welding arc. The casualty complains of a painful eye

Eye irrigation   Tilt the casualty's head to one side and direct the flow of water from the nose down over the injured eye, preventing contamination of the good eye. The eye should be held open if necessary.

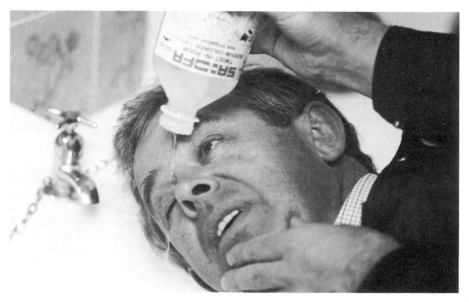

some hours after looking at the bright light and usually feels that there are several foreign bodies in it. On examination (see under 'Foreign Bodies in the Eye' previously) the white part of the eye appears inflamed, but no foreign bodies can be seen. The condition will resolve within twenty-four hours if the casualty is placed in a dark room and reassured. Medical advice should be sought in case the diagnosis is incorrect.

Arc eye can be prevented by wearing protective goggles when welding. Arc eye generally occurs in people watching welding operations rather than in welders themselves, who know the value of wearing protective goggles.

Poisoning

The list of poisonous substances which are used in various parts of the oil and gas processing system grows longer every day. The precise mode of action and antidotes to each of these substances is a specialized subject outside the scope of this book, and in any case does not affect the immediate care of the poisoned casualty.

How poisons act
A poison is a substance which interferes with the functions of the body cells. Its ultimate effect on the body depends on the dose and the length of time it is in contact with the cells. Given time, the body will either excrete or change most poisonous substances to an inactive form. Provided the basic functions of the body can be maintained, such as supplying oxygen to the cells, the body can recover from most cases of poisoning. The poison may enter the body in several ways:

- By inhalation, for example exhaust fumes from a compressor, or other toxic gases (see Chapter 8)
- By swallowing, for example food poisoning (see Chapter 10) or the accidental swallowing of chemicals
- By absorption through the skin, for example epoxy resins which are used in the repair of concrete underwater structures
- By injection through the skin, for example by dangerous marine life, snakes and accidentally or deliberately by means of a syringe.

How you treat a case of poisoning depends not on the type of poison but on the method by which it entered the body, such as inhalation or swallowing.

Poisoning by inhalation
This is dealt with in Chapter 8.

Food poisoning
This is dealt with in Chapter 10.

Treatment of an unconscious casualty who has swallowed poison

1. If the casualty is already unconscious when found he should be placed in the recovery position. He should have medical help.
2. If poisoning is suspected and the poison is available a specimen of it should be sent to hospital with the casualty.
3. No attempt should ever be made to give anything by mouth to an unconscious casualty or to make him sick. Doing either of these things is likely to kill him.
4. Since the dose of poison taken is not known the patient must be watched carefully. He may regain consciousness or become more deeply unconscious; his breathing and then his heart may stop. You must be prepared to give resuscitation treatment if necessary (see pages 31–9).

Treatment of a conscious casualty who has swallowed poison

1. When the conscious casualty complains of having taken a poison by mouth it is important immediately to determine whether it is corrosive or not. If it is not corrosive proceed to step 4 below. If it is corrosive the casualty will tell you because it will have burned his mouth, he will be in great pain and there will be burn marks around his lips and mouth. Common corrosive poisons include caustic soda and sulphuric acid.

    The oesophagus connecting the mouth to the stomach is thin-walled and very vulnerable. If it is perforated by a corrosive substance the casualty will become very seriously ill and may die. Under these circumstances, give the casualty a bland fluid to drink. This washes out the oesophagus and dilutes the corrosive substance in the stomach.

    Milk is probably the best fluid, but do not waste time looking for it, water will do just as well.
2. Do not make the casualty sick, because if he vomits, the burning which occurred as he swallowed the poison will happen again as he regurgitates it.
3. If the poison is non-corrosive – an overdose of drugs, for example – then try to make the casualty sick. This will reduce the dose of poison available to be absorbed from the bowel into the bloodstream. The best way to do this is to place your fingers at the back of the casualty's throat. Do not give salty drinks, they do

Opposite: Flow chart showing the steps to take when a casualty has swallowed poison.

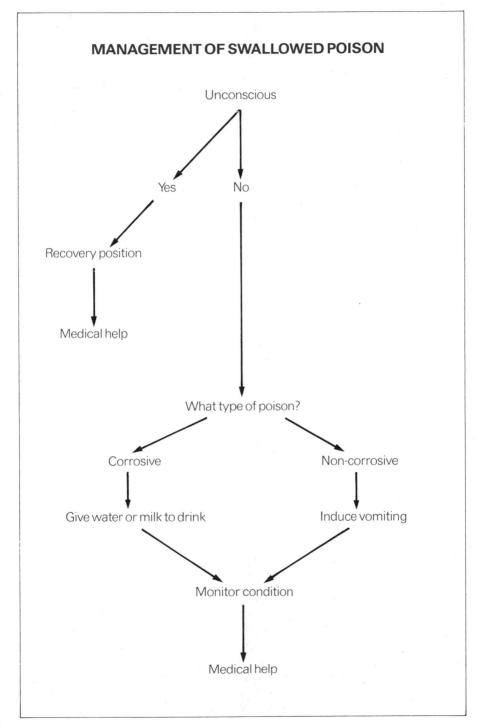

MANAGEMENT OF SWALLOWED POISON

Unconscious

Yes   No

Recovery position

Medical help

What type of poison?

Corrosive   Non-corrosive

Give water or milk to drink   Induce vomiting

Monitor condition

Medical help

not always cause vomiting and can make the condition worse. Bland fluids can then be given and the casualty can be made sick a second time in order to get rid of as much poison as possible. Transfer him to hospital urgently remembering to take a specimen of the poison or the vomit or the empty bottle which contained the poison.

4. It is very important that the person escorting the poisoned casualty to hospital is skilled in first aid. He should be able to monitor the casualty so that he can take action should the casualty become unconscious, or his breathing or heart stop (see pages 31–9 and 119).

Poisoning by skin absorption
This is caused by substances such as mercury and epoxy resins. It results in slowly developing illnesses for which there is no specific first aid. If poisoning by skin absorption is suspected medical advice should be sought.

Poisoning by injection
The principles of managing a casualty with an injected poison are basically the same whether it is a snake bite, the wrong dose of a drug or a poison injected by means of a syringe.

1. Injected poison cannot be sucked out.
2. Injected poison may be absorbed slowly.
3. The best immediate care is to transfer the casualty as quickly as possible to specialist medical help. Remember to take a specimen of the poison or the animal or a description of the animal.
4. The casualty must be monitored while he is being transferred to hospital (see page 119). He may become unconscious or his breathing or heart may stop. Appropriate resuscitation should be taken in these circumstances (see pages 31–9). If you can get the casualty to hospital alive, his life may well be saved even though he may have been bitten by a very poisonous snake.

Snake bites and fish stings   All sea snakes are poisonous, as are several species of fish. In hot areas of the world many offshore personnel, especially divers, have been bitten or stung by them. Snake bites and fish stings tend to cause the most tremendous panic. It is very important to avoid actions which will cause more harm than good, such as trying to suck out the poison. The priority is to get the casualty to hospital as quickly as possible. It may be helpful to reassure him that venom is normally injected by snakes or fish only as a means of paralysing their prey or supply of foodstuff, not in defence. Even the most toxic snake will not always inject venom. In 60 per cent of snake bite cases there is little evidence to show that venom has been injected. Even if venom *is* injected, reports are increasing of survival from the bite of even the most poisonous snakes, provided the casualty is transferred rapidly and efficiently to hospital by experienced first aiders.

Identification of the snake or fish type can be helpful – if it has been killed take it with you, but don't waste time if it hasn't, the casualty needs hospital care quickly; there is nothing you can do apart from getting him there. Remember he may stop breathing or his heart may stop beating on the journey to hospital, so be ready to give resuscitation if necessary (see Chapter 3).

5. HANDLING THE CASUALTY

Once a casualty's survival has been secured by emergency life support and his injuries treated with appropriate first aid, the next step is to move him away from the site of the accident to the sick bay, and eventually, if advised by the rig medic or doctor, to the helideck for transportation ashore. Casualty handling and offshore transportation are the subjects of the next two chapters.

The golden rule in casualty handling is that a casualty should not be moved until there is a good reason to do so. If the casualty is in a life-threatening situation he must be moved immediately without any time for further assessment. Some examples of this would be:

- A casualty in a toxic atmosphere, for example, following an escape of hydrogen sulphide gas (see Chapter 8)
- In the presence of fire, for example, following a blow-out
- A casualty who has become unconscious and has severe bleeding from the mouth, for example, following a blow to the head from a crane hook (see Chapter 4).

It is important to move the casualty only as far as is necessary to remove him from the life-threatening situation. In the case of the unconscious casualty bleeding from the mouth, moving him onto his side is all that is required.

If no life-threatening situation exists, the casualty should be assessed carefully and examined before he is moved. During examination, injuries such as fractures of the lower limb will be discovered and should be immobilized before the casualty is moved (see Chapter 4).

The move should be carefully planned, bearing the following factors in mind:

1. The type of immobilization the casualty requires.
2. The type of lift or stretcher to be used (see later in this chapter).
3. Where the casualty should be moved to: to the sick bay, for example, or to the sick bay and then the helideck.
4. The quickest and/or safest route to use.

It is important to remember that non-emergency moves should be carried out in such a way that additional injury does not occur and the casualty is not caused discomfort or pain. For example, following a crush injury to the abdomen there may be internal bleeding. Blood generally clots so the bleeding may stop spontaneously. But clumsy handling of the casualty may cause the clots to dislodge, restarting the bleeding.

It is possible to move a casualty either by assisting or lifting, or by using a stretcher.

Assisting or lifting

Only the table of knees lift described on pages 106–8 protects the casualty's spine or provides adequate protection for unsplinted fractures.

In an emergency use the most effective of the methods described below for the amount of time available to move the casualty. The rescuer must himself take care not to injure his back. You should bend from the knees and keep a straight back to avoid unnecessary back strain.

Lifts for one rescuer

One-rescuer assist is suitable when the casualty is conscious and can walk with assistance. Standing at the casualty's injured side (unless he has an injured arm) put your arm round his waist and grasp his clothing at the hip. Put his arm round your neck and hold his hand with your free hand (see overleaf).

Piggy-back carry This is a standard piggy-back and is suitable when the casualty is conscious, can stand and has no fractures of the extremities (see overleaf).

Fireman's lift is suitable with conscious or unconscious casualties who do not have fractures of the extremities. This lift is best used on lightweight casualties (see overleaf).

1. Help the casualty into an upright position facing you.
2. Take his right wrist with your left hand.
3. Bend down putting your head under his extended right arm until your right shoulder is level with the lower part of his abdomen.
4. Put your right arm between his legs.
5. Stand up taking his weight onto your right shoulder.

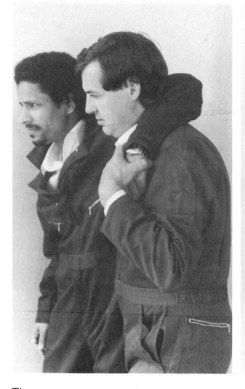

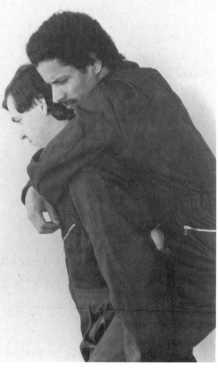

The one-rescuer assist may be all that is necessary to help move a conscious casualty who can walk.

A piggy-back carry is simple and can be effective in an emergency. It can be used for a conscious casualty.

6. Pull the casualty across your shoulders and transfer his right wrist to your right hand.

One-rescuer drags can be used for the conscious or unconscious casualty. They work best on a smooth surface. The casualty should be lying on his back. Straddle the casualty, facing towards him, and get him to clasp you round the neck. Crawl forward. If he is unconscious, tie his wrists together and loop them over your head. Except in the direst emergency these drags are unsuitable for casualties with a broken hand, wrist, arm or shoulder.

1
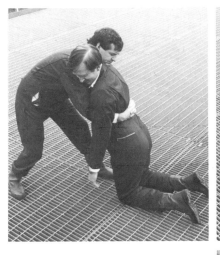

2
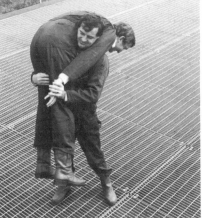

3
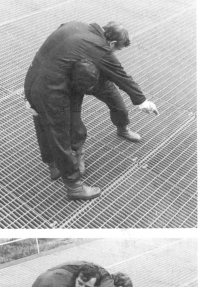

Fireman's lift

1. Help the casualty into an upright position, facing you.

2. Take the casualty's right wrist with your left hand. Bend down, putting your head under his extended right arm and put your right arm between or around his legs.

3. Carefully stand up taking his weight onto your right shoulder. Pull the casualty across your shoulders and transfer his right wrist to your right hand.

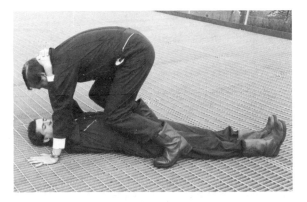

It is possible to drag a conscious casualty away from danger by getting him to clasp his hands around your neck. You can then crawl forward taking the casualty with you.

Lifts for two rescuers

Four-handed seat   This method is used to carry a conscious casualty who can assist the bearers by using one or both arms to hold on.

1. The two rescuers face each other behind the casualty.
2. They grasp their own left wrists with their right hands and the other rescuer's right wrist with their left hand.
3. They stoop behind the casualty who places an arm round each rescuer's neck and raises himself to sit on the four-handed seat.

Two-handed seat   This method is used to carry a casualty who is unable to assist the bearers.

1. The two rescuers face each other and stoop each side of the casualty.
2. Each rescuer passes his arm nearest the casualty round the casualty's back just below the shoulders and holds some clothing.
3. They pass their other arms under the casualty's thighs and clasp hands with the hook grip.

Four-handed seat
The two rescuers should form a strong seat with their arms, as described in the text above, and stoop behind the casualty ready to pick him up.

2. Rear view of a four-handed seat.

2

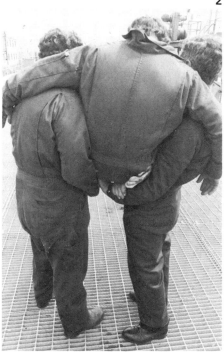

1

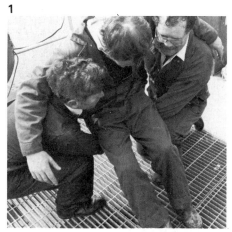

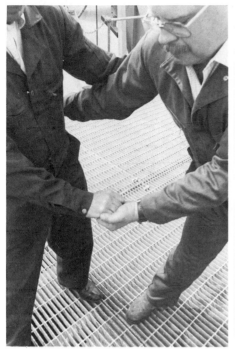

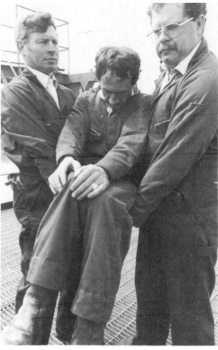

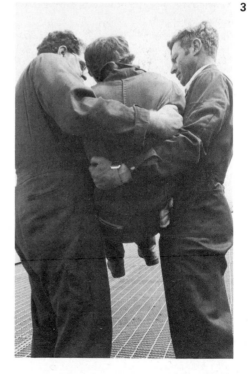

Two-handed seat
1. Hand grip for a two-handed seat.

2. The two-handed seat should be used to carry a casualty who is unable to assist the bearers.

3. Rear view of a two-handed seat, showing the supportive clasp of the bearers across the back of the casualty.

4. For the hook grip the rescuer on the left of the patient has his palm upwards with his fingers bent up. The other rescuer hooks his hand into this with his palm downwards and fingers bent down. It may be more comfortable to hold a handkerchief between the two hands to prevent damage with the finger nails.

Handling a casualty with suspected spinal injury
Damage to the spinal cord with consequent permanent paralysis is such a terrible consequence of clumsy handling of a casualty with a back injury that extra special care must be taken when attending to this type of injury. The possibility of back injury must be suspected:

- Following a fall from a height
- In multiple injuries
- When back pain is complained of
- Following a 'jack-knife' type of injury, for example where the casualty's body has been sharply bent against a bulkhead.

Remember that the signs of a back injury may sometimes seem insignificant – but the possibility must always be borne in mind.

There is no hurry to move such a casualty. If he must be moved, carefully plan in advance the means of moving him out and if necessary practise the lift or move with a healthy subject first. The principle is to avoid all movements of the spine during the move, bearing in mind that twisting movement is more likely to cause serious injury than see-sawing. It is not necessary to fit a spinal splint before moving a casualty with a suspected spinal injury.

The table of knees lift   The aluminium scoop stretcher (see pages 111–12) is the best and safest method of moving a casualty with a suspected back injury to a stretcher suitable for transportation. If a scoop stretcher is not available the next best method is to use the table of knees lift. For this four men are needed and they should practise the lift several times with a healthy subject before attempting to move the casualty. The technique is as follows (see illustrations opposite):

1. Three men kneel alongside the casualty and each man raises one knee – either right or left, but it should be the same knee for each lifter.
2. The lifters' arms are placed under the body of the casualty and the man in charge of the lift places himself on the other side.
3. It is vital that the lift should be precisely coordinated, so the man in charge should ask, 'Are you ready?' On being given a positive response from all, he shall then give the word of command, 'Lift.'

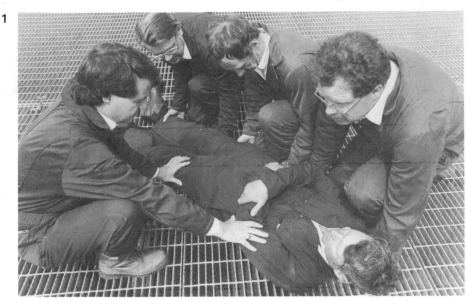

The table of knees lift

1. Three lifters should be positioned on one side of the casualty, one lifter on the other.

2. Support the casualty on the table of knees formed by the three lifters on one side of the body until the fourth man has placed the stretcher in position.

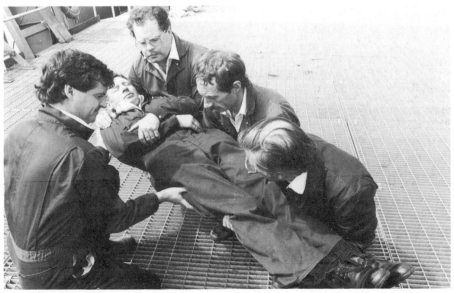

4. The casualty is then lifted onto the table of knees, the man in charge assisting with the heavy head and chest end.
5. When the man in charge is satisfied that the casualty is held in a stable position he should move off and place the stretcher in front of the men holding the casualty.
6. From the other side of the stretcher the man in charge of the lift shall then coordinate the lowering procedure by using the commands, 'Are you ready to lower?' and on receiving an affirmative response, 'Lower.'
7. The lifting team should then lower the casualty as slowly and smoothly as possible onto the stretcher.

Stretchers

These are the easiest and safest methods of transport for casualties who are unable to walk, or who have an injury which may be aggravated by unnecessary movement. Stretchers can be used to carry a casualty away from the site of an accident to the sick bay, and later to the helideck. They are also useful for installation-to-ship transfer and vice versa.

Several types of stretcher are now available and if used correctly they can be invaluable. All offshore installations will have at least one of the types described in this section. The simple pole and canvas stretcher is not very suitable in the offshore environment. It does not protect the casualty's spine and cannot be used to transport casualties vertically.

Neill Robertson stretcher

This is made of stout canvas and bamboo. This stretcher is designed for lifting casualties in the upright position through small hatches or for hoisting or lowering casualties from heights. When the casualty is placed on the stretcher, the strap at the top is passed around his forehead to hold his head in position. The upper flaps are wrapped around the casualty's chest and secured with two short straps, leaving the arms outside. The casualty's arms are then secured with the long strap. The lower straps are secured around the lower limbs. The ring at the head of the stretcher is used for hoisting. A length of rope is attached to the ring at the foot of the stretcher to guide the stretcher during hoisting.

The stretcher should be stored where it is most likely to be needed – in the sick bay, near the drill floor and near the helideck, for instance – together with a suitable length of rope (made of a rot-proof fibre), and should be available at each level of the installation. The drawbacks of the Neill Robertson stretcher are that it is liable to rot, particularly

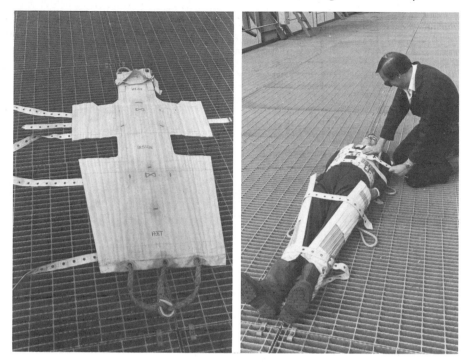

Neill Robertson stretcher
1. Lay out the stretcher as shown ready for use.

2. Lay the casualty on the stretcher and secure the flaps of the stretcher firmly around his body by tying down the straps.

in the salt atmosphere found off shore and must therefore be checked frequently. It is also too small to deal with a casualty over 6 ft (2 m) in height. Also, this stretcher will bend, so great care must be taken when dealing with a casualty who has a possible back injury.

Paraguard stretcher
This is similar to the Neill Robertson stretcher and is used for the same purpose (see overleaf). It is much more expensive but has the following advantages over the Neill Robertson stretcher.

1. It is more easily carried as it can be packed away in its rucksack.
2. It is more durable and reliable for lifting.
3. It is ideal for a casualty with a back injury because it has a reinforced back.
4. It can be hoisted horizontally as well as vertically.
5. It can bend in the middle to negotiate obstacles.
6. It is longer and more suitable for a tall (over 6 ft/1.8 m) casualty.

1

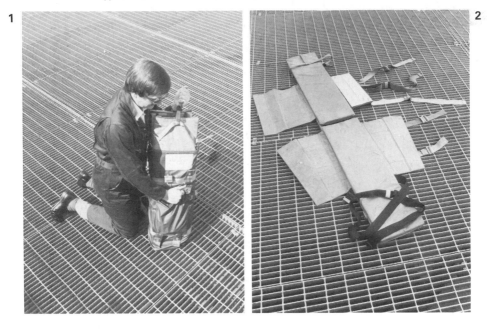

2

3

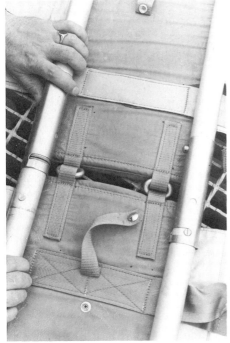

Paraguard stretcher
1. This stretcher comes in a convenient weatherproof backpack.

2. Lay out the pieces of stretcher as
shown.

3. The stretcher is not secure and
safe to use until the brackets have
been fixed. Slide them over the pole
joints and twist to secure them over
the buttons, as has been done with
the right-hand bracket in the
photograph.

4

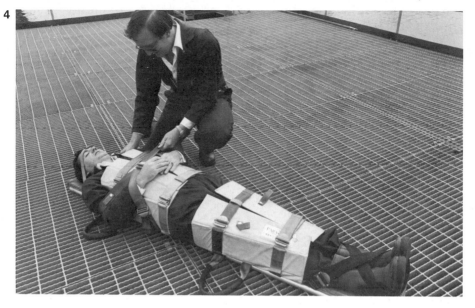

4. Lie the casualty on the stretcher and fold the sides up and over the body. Secure with straps provided.

Aluminium scoop stretcher

The scoop, or orthopaedic stretcher, is an adjustable stretcher used to lift casualties with minimum movement of the spine (see overleaf). It is therefore excellent for picking up someone with a suspected fracture of the spine or internal injuries.

The casualty needs to be flat on his back. Separate the stretcher into its two parts, one on either side of the casualty, and connect it at the top above his head. Then scoop it together under the casualty with a gentle side-to-side motion, moving him as little as possible.

Although the length of the stretcher can be adjusted to suit any size of casualty, it is not a very safe or comfortable rescue stretcher. When the casualty has been picked up using the scoop stretcher, he can be transferred immediately to another stretcher (e.g. the paraguard stretcher) which is more suitable for rescue.

Basket-type stretcher

These are usually made of wire or plastic and can be hoisted horizontally. It has patient security straps and an adjustable foot-rest to provide additional security.

This is the most comfortable of all stretchers and ideally suited for transporting the patient in a helicopter. But it is a large stretcher which

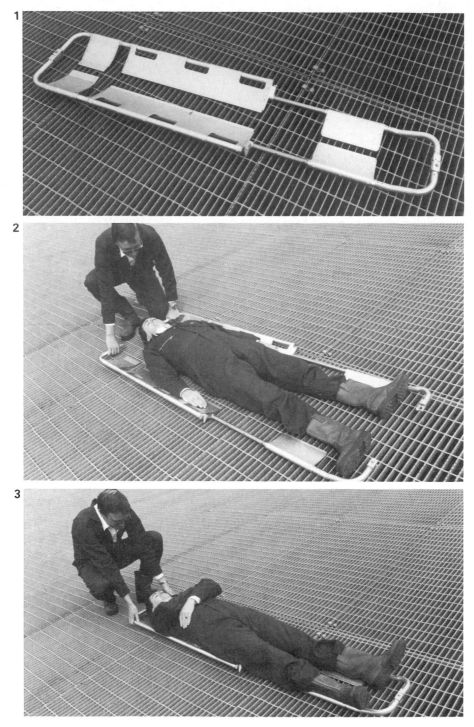

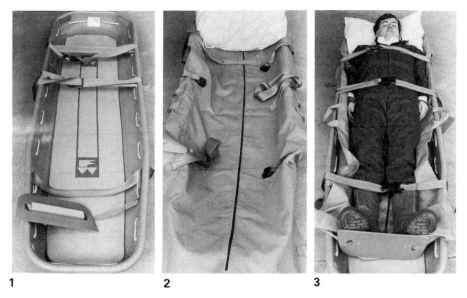

1   2   3

Basket-type stretcher (*above*)
1. The stretcher, showing the securing straps and adjustable foot board.

2. A casualty should never be placed into the basket stretcher unless a canvas sheet or blanket has been positioned in the bottom of the stretcher so he can be removed easily from the stretcher.

3. Lay the casualty in position on the blanket with the foot board attached and secure the straps across the body.

is not suitable for a rescue operation, being too cumbersome. Because of the high sides on this stretcher, a casualty should never be placed in it unless a canvas sheet or blanket is under him which can be used to remove him from the stretcher. This stretcher can fill with water, so, if necessary, measures should be taken to avoid this happening.

Vacuum mattress
This is a new type of stretcher consisting of a durable material covering a mass of small, expanded polystyrene pellets. The casualty can be put

Aluminium scoop stretcher (*opposite*)
1. The length of this stretcher can be adjusted to fit the casualty, the wider end of the stretcher being the head end.

2. The stretcher splits into two parts lengthwise. These can then be positioned either side of the casualty and 'scooped' under him.

3. Join the two halves of the stretcher together with the casualty in position. The stretcher is now ready for use.

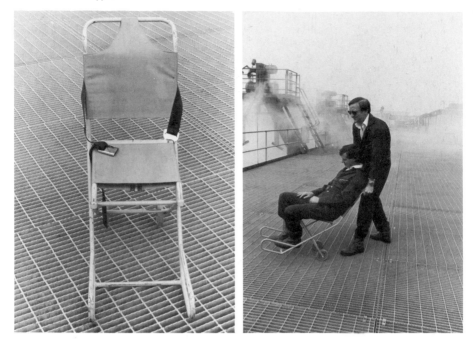

Folding stair chair
This chair can be used to wheel a casualty along a flat surface or to lift him down steps.

The folding stair chair in use on a flat surface.

onto this mattress and when air is evacuated the stretcher goes rigid and forms a mould around his body.

The vacuum mattress is good for casualties with multiple injuries; being the equivalent of a full body splint, it will prevent unnecessary movement. It is also useful for moving unconscious casualties, because it is easy to place someone on a vacuum mattress in the recovery position.

Folding stair chair

Most models have two rear leg wheels. Stair chairs are useful when transferring a casualty downstairs or through narrow spaces. These devices are not recommended for use with unconscious or disoriented casualties.

Blanket lift

In a desperate situation where a casualty needs to be moved urgently and there is no stretcher immediately available, as might be the case

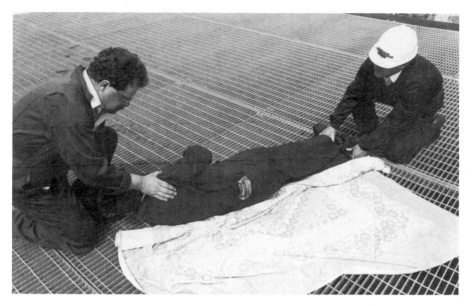

The blanket lift
1. Turn the casualty gently onto his side and tuck the rolled part of the blanket against his back.

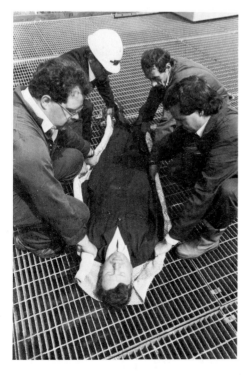

2. Turn the casualty onto the other side and unroll the blanket from underneath him. To lift the casualty, roll up the edges of the blanket against the sides of the body and lift gently.

following a multicasualty accident, a stretcher can be improvized using a blanket. If there is time test the blanket lift on a healthy colleague before attempting to lift the injured man.

To place a blanket under the casualty roll the blanket lengthwise for half its width and place the roll in line with and against the casualty. Then gently turn him onto his side without bending his neck or twisting his body. The rolled part of the blanket is then moved against the casualty's back. He is gently turned back over the roll onto his opposite side. The blanket is unrolled and the casualty is gently turned onto his back.

To lift the blanket, roll the edges up against the sides of the casualty and lift them gently.

Summary of casualty handling
1. The casualty should not be moved at all unless there is a good reason.
2. He may have to be moved in an emergency if his life is threatened.
3. If he has to be moved the most efficient method that time permits must be used.
4. If no life-threatening situation exists, the casualty should be assessed and examined by the rescuer before he is moved.
5. First-aid treatment should be given. Any fractures should be immobilized. Then the movement of the casualty should be planned.
6. Careful and skilful casualty handling and transportation are very important to prevent further injuries being caused.

The problems do not end when the casualty has been successfully loaded into the helicopter or ship, for he still has a long way to go to hospital. This phase of management is dealt with in the next chapter.

6. TRANSPORTATION OFFSHORE

The helicopter is now the normal means of transport to and from offshore installations both for routine crew changes as well as for the injured and sick.

The noise and vibration in most helicopters may cause stress and fatigue on a long journey and some form of ear protection must be worn. This is particularly important for a day trip when the journey to and from the offshore installation is made in one day. Ear protectors will preserve efficiency following a helicopter journey and protect the hearing of those who travel frequently by helicopter.

Transporting casualties by helicopter

Helicopter transport enables a sick or injured man to be taken from the offshore structure straight to the hospital onshore. A casualty can be plucked or winched from the sea, the deck of a ship or an offshore structure. Or if the helicopter can land on the helideck of the offshore structure the casualty can be carefully placed inside it.

The casualty must be in a stable condition before the journey begins. The journey may take several hours, so he will require continuing attention during the journey. For this reason most oil companies train a group of offshore personnel to provide an escort service for casualties (see page 21).

Assessing transportation priorities
In most oil and gas field developments a certain number of helicopters are constantly available for transporting medical emergencies. If it is necessary to transport more casualties than can be done with the helicopter facilities immediately available it is necessary to decide which casualties to evacuate first. Paradoxically, it is not always appropriate to evacuate the more seriously ill casualties first.

For example, following a fire there may be a number of seriously burned casualties who have been treated as recommended (see pages 86–91). Suppose there are six burned patients awaiting evacuation.

They have burns involving the following percentage areas of body surface: 9, 31, 40, 45, 80, 85 respectively. If the helicopter can only take three patients the problem is to decide who should be sent ashore first. It should be the three patients whose burned surface is 31, 40 and 45 per cent, because they are at risk of dying if they do not receive medical attention urgently but have a good chance of survival if they receive hospital attention. The casualties with burned surfaces of 80 and 85 per cent will probably die whether they receive medical attention or not. While the casualty whose burn amounts to 9 per cent of his body surface needs medical attention, but his condition will not get worse if he has to wait for the next helicopter.

Consider another scenario, this time in the Arabian summer. Following an accident, a number of minor injuries are caused which require hospital attention. One casualty also has a badly crushed chest and is in shock, and another is suffering from severe heat stroke. A medical team arrives in a helicopter and a second helicopter is expected to arrive within the hour. On this occasion it is the patients with minor injuries who should go on the first helicopter, while the medical team resuscitate the two seriously injured casualties. These two can then be accompanied by the medical team in the second helicopter in a stable condition. Under these circumstances the seriously injured men are more likely to withstand the journey.

Preparing for evacuation
If the casualty has to be evacuated the following actions can be taken while waiting for the helicopter:

1. **Escort**   It may be better if the rig medic does not escort the patient ashore, because the remaining personnel on the rig would be left with no medical assistance. Therefore a suitable escort should be chosen, preferably someone with basic life support training.
2. **Monitoring** of the patient should continue while waiting for transport and during the journey (see opposite). The escort should be instructed on what to do and the problems which might arise.
3. **An account** of the incident should be written down, if it has not been done before, with times of the various events noted. This should be sent ashore with the casualty.
4. **No food or drink** should be given to the casualty because he may have to have an anaesthetic during later treatment. Exceptions to this general rule of no fluids are burns victims and casualties in hot climates who may be at risk of dehydration (see Chapter 7).
5. **Additional evidence** which might be of value to the hospital team, such as a bottle or chemical specimen if there is suspected poisoning, should be sent ashore with the patient. Or if he has

vomited, any contaminated clothing or vomit should also be sent with him.

These procedures are vital to the continuing management of the patient. Seeing them being performed he will also feel more confident and reassured while waiting for the helicopter to arrive.

Monitoring the casualty in flight

We have already stressed the importance of monitoring a casualty continuously during the journey. With the escort's notes and verbal account of the trip the hospital doctor receiving the casualty can begin treatment at once without spending an unnecessary amount of time determining the patient's condition.

Monitoring the casualty can be very difficult in a helicopter with all the noise and vibration. There have been occasions when casualties have been plucked from the sea and it has been hard to distinguish between life and death in the noisy environment of the helicopter. In certain cases special equipment can be used to measure vital signs visually, where auditory means are more usual – determining the presence of a heartbeat or measuring blood pressure, for instance. Standard monitoring equipment which functions well in a helicopter is also available – for example, some types of electrocardiogram (ECG) for measuring heart activity.

During the journey the attendant must make sure that the casualty is breathing and his heart is beating. Any bleeding should be kept under control and fractures and wounds should be kept immobilized (see Chapters 3 and 4). It is also important to monitor changes in the patient's condition in case it deteriorates and he needs more treatment. For example, when escorting a casualty who has been poisoned his breathing may stop. If artificial respiration can be given before the heart stops, he will have a good chance of survival (see pages 31–5). Or, a splint immobilizing a fracture may become too tight and hinder the circulation if there is further swelling at the fracture site. It will then need to be loosened.

Communication

Before the helicopter reaches the offshore casualty the doctor on board may have to contact the first aider or medic on the offshore structure. The person escorting the casualty back to shore may also have to contact the medical centre or hospital onshore. For example, if the casualty is getting worse, special facilities may be needed at the heliport to deal with him.

This communication is not easy because radio equipment does not allow free discussion and reception may be poor. Therefore short, relevant messages about the casualty's condition should be used (see pages 53–4). Communicating in this way may need practice, which should be obtained before an emergency arises.

Other forms of transportation for casualties

Boats can also be used to transfer the injured or to convey a member of the onshore health care team to the scene of the accident. Sometimes the casualty may get his injury on board a boat. Transport by boat takes longer than helicopter travel but the journey may be smoother and less noisy.

If a member of the health care team travels by boat to the offshore structure he will be transferred to the structure rather than having the casualty transferred to the boat. This is done by using a special type of basket which can transfer him from the heaving deck to and from the installation, which may be up to 150 ft (45 m) above.

If a man is injured on board a boat it may be best to steam to the nearest port for onshore treatment. If his condition is serious he may be winched aboard a helicopter and taken ashore. Where possible a

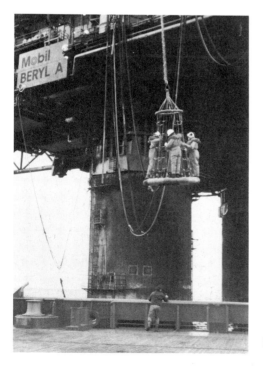

Ship to rig transfer by basket.

medic or paramedic should visit him first to determine what care is needed and to prepare him for helicopter transfer if necessary.

If the diver in a saturation chamber becomes ill and he is diving from a ship, it can steam for port. But this is not possible if the pressure chambers are mounted on a fixed offshore installation (see Chapter 9). If transfer to a sophisticated hyperbaric facility is necessary, a transfer system to maintain the diver at the same atmospheric pressure is needed – a hyperbaric lifeboat, for example, or a series of transfer chambers as used at Aberdeen (see pages 158–60).

Installation abandonment

In the event of a major disaster offshore, such as a rig fire, the offshore installation manager or his deputy may decide to evacuate all personnel. The usual means of abandoning an installation is by lifeboat, and everyone working offshore must be familiar with the installation's own particular lifeboat drill. In a disaster situation, there may not be time to administer all the necessary first aid to casualties, or to place them in stretchers before getting them into the lifeboats. All that can be done is to take as much care with them as is allowed by the circumstances.

In the British sector of the North Sea it is a legal requirement for a standby boat to be available to assist survivors.

An enclosed lifeboat taking part in an abandonment exercise.

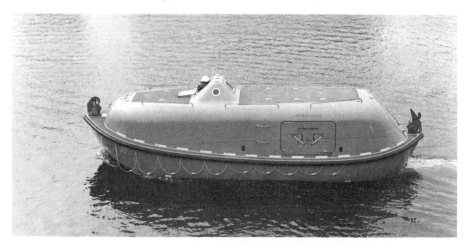

Helicopter ditching

The health and safety problems related to offshore transportation are not confined to escorting the injured or sick back onshore for medical treatment. All offshore personnel are at risk of becoming casualties themselves in the course of routine helicopter travel between the mainland and the installation. Fortunately the number of helicopter ditchings is small. At the time of writing there are approximately 100 helicopters in use in the North Sea, the frequency of ditching being around one ditching every two years. During 1977, for example 350,000 passengers were carried to and from the heliports of mainland Scotland and the offshore installations in the northern North Sea. The average daily passenger load in 1984 was 1,000 people. However, helicopter ditching is more common than a crash in a fixed-wing aircraft.

The Sikorski helicopters were designed to float following a controlled ditching, giving passengers time to enter a survival capsule and await rescue. But this only happens in very calm conditions, with a low swell. Usually during a ditching the rotor blade contacts a high wave and the helicopter turns over.

The problems which have to be faced following a helicopter ditching are:

1. Getting out of the helicopter.
2. Combating drowning and hypothermia.
3. Entering a survival capsule.
4. Staying alive.

Getting out of the helicopter
When a helicopter ditches the passengers may panic. If the helicopter turns upside down they may also be confused and disorientated. Passengers should practise leaving a ditched helicopter before they travel. The Offshore Survival Centre at Aberdeen's Robert Gordon's Institute of Technology has designed a simple machine which simulates ditching and gives the students practice at leaving an enclosed space.

When it becomes likely that the helicopter will ditch, or after it has ditched (depending on the time available for preparation and on the instructions of the air crew), if survival suits are worn they must be closed up and made ready for use. The lifejacket is normally worn over the survival suit and tied round the waist. It must now be opened out and placed over the head. Do not inflate the jacket because it may make emerging from the helicopter difficult if it is inflated.

If the helicopter does not turn over, it may be possible to launch the life raft and pull in the painter so that the passengers can step across into the water. If the helicopter turns over it is important that you should already have identified the exit, because you will be disorientated. If you are sitting close to a door put your hand on the handle. If the nearest exit is two seats in front point your hand at it and keep pointing. Wait for the cabin to fill with water before attempting to open the exit. When the door is open, leave the helicopter and then inflate the lifejacket.

Combating drowning and hypothermia

When a helicopter ditches in a cold part of the world and the passengers manage to escape from the cabin their next problem is to prevent drowning (see detailed discussion on pages 144–5) and cooling of the body, or hypothermia (see detailed discussion on pages 134–8).

For example, in the northern North Sea seasonal variation in water temperature is 40–54°F (5–12°C) and the average monthly wind velocity is 15–35 kt. Without some form of protective clothing death from hypothermia or drowning will occur in approximately half an hour.

The airway of a man floating in sea water wearing an inflated, standard lifejacket is only about 0.4 ft (0.15 m) above the water surface. A victim may ride the large, regularly curved waves but short steep seas and choppy waves will break over his head. For example, the average wave height in the northern North Sea has been shown to exceed 1.6 ft (0.5 m) for 98 per cent of the year. To make matters worse a man in the water will automatically be turned to face the wind spray, because his body acts as a sea-anchor in the water. Thus, he can drown without being submerged if he loses control of his breathing because of wave splash, surface turbulence and sea sickness.

Factors which increase the risk of hypothermia are:

- Excessive or unnecessary movement in the water
- Lack of body fat
- Increased age
- Insufficient garments worn under protective clothing
- Lack of recent food intake
- Recent alcohol intake.

Factors which increase the risk of drowning are:

- Lack of buoyancy aids
- Fatigue and exhaustion
- Disorientation and lack of muscle coordination
- Lack of physical fitness
- Lack of emergency drill practice
- Associated burns and other injuries.

Survival suits   To combat hypothermia, passenger survival suits are now available in Britain for passengers and crew during helicopter travel over water.

All types of survival suit should guarantee the wearer immersed in still water at 40°F (5°C) at least one to two hours of protection against the onset of hypothermia.

The suits are designed to fit over normal clothing, but not being tailored they fit poorly. Some makers produce large, medium and small sizes. Nowadays the dry suit is most commonly used. It maintains relative dryness by having tight seals around the face and the wrists and it has integral feet covering. There is a problem in the distribution of retained air within the suit, which may affect the orientation of the body in water, particularly if large quantities of air are retained around the legs. At worst, this air can force the wearer upside down in the water! Valves are fitted to counter this problem, but they are not very efficient and may let water in.

A wet suit is made of similar waterproof material, and fits over the clothing like an extra protective suit, but water can enter freely at the neck and wrists. It is tucked into the boots and does not include integral feet covering. Such garments have been shown at times to contain many gallons of water in the trousers alone, trapped there by the boots, and so cannot be considered as safe as the dry suits.

Survival suits are normally handed out at the heliport. The operating company often employs a service company to issue them and ensure that they are maintained in a good state of repair. The suits are normally returned on arrival at the offshore installation and are re-issued when it is time to leave. Individual workers do not pay for the hire of suits and the type of suit worn is a matter of company policy.

Lifejackets are still required to provide buoyancy and a correct angle of flotation in the water. Survival suits are not designed to give correct buoyancy therefore the lifejacket must fit over the survival suit.

Entering a survival capsule

Getting into a survival capsule may be easy if the helicopter has not turned over and the painter can be pulled to the entrance. Passengers can then step across into the capsule without entering the water. But usually it is not easy to enter a survival capsule, particularly if it is moving, the sea is rough and you are exhausted and weighed down with a protective suit and boots. Entering a capsule is more difficult if there is much retained air in the dry suit, and nearly impossible if there is a considerable pool of water in the wet suit or a leak in the dry suit which has allowed water to seep in.

Entry will also be difficult if the man in the water has hypothermia

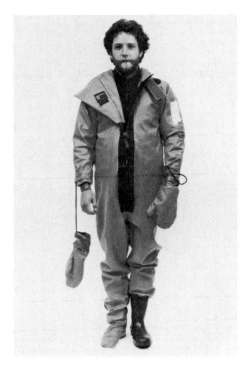

A dry suit currently in use on North
Sea rigs.

(see pages 134–8), because it will limit his muscle coordination and
cloud his judgement and intellectual function. Practice in entering
survival capsules is essential and can be obtained at the various onshore
survival schools.

The main problems when the passenger is in the water are caused
by the drag of the survival suit and the inflated lip, or sponson, at the
entrance to the capsule. The problem is greatest for the first man, but
there is a rope in the capsule which he can use to help himself aboard.
The second man can be helped in by the first man. When the first two
are in the capsule they should position themselves on each side of the
entrance and assist the remaining passengers in. Usually the remaining
passengers are helped in backwards over the sponson. Some survival
suits have a hook on the back which can be used to help lift the
passenger into the capsule.

Staying alive
Survival capsules are normally enclosed to protect the occupants from
waves, very hot and cold temperatures and wind chill. For example,
at an air temperature of 59°F (15°C) a wind velocity of 20–30 kt

would produce a cooling effect on exposed flesh similar to that at −11°F (−24°C) with no wind.

It is important that the water should be kept out of the capsule because wetting greatly inceases the rate of heat loss. When the capsule has been sealed the occupants should keep dry and try to change into dry garments if they are available.

If food is available in the capsule, it should be eaten because it is a useful means of maintaining body heat.

Another problem in bad weather is sea sickness. If one man is sick the others may become sick, which makes conditions in the capsule extremely unpleasant. But, because of the dangers of wind exposure it is important not to open the flap to reduce the smell.

If the ditching occurs during a routine flight from an offshore structure the survivors will generally be rescued quickly and the time spent waiting in the survival capsule will not be long.

In the next chapter we examine in more detail the problems caused by cold − and heat − and how to combat them.

7. PROBLEMS CAUSED BY HEAT AND COLD

Many oil and gas reserves are situated in remote areas of the world which are inaccessible and either very hot, such as the Arabian Gulf or the Gulf of Mexico, or very cold, such as Alaska or the North Sea. These extreme temperatures in association with wind speed and humidity can cause injury to offshore workers exposed to the elements.

In cold areas a high wind speed increases the cooling effect on man. Temperature and wind velocity are closely associated and can be related in the wind-chill scale (see overleaf). The lower the temperature and the greater the wind velocity the greater is the cooling effect.

On the other hand, high wind speeds in very hot areas are beneficial, as they increase cooling by moving air laden with moisture from the surface of the body, and allow sweat to evaporate. In hot climates, though, high humidity limits your ability to sweat and regulate your body temperature. And in cold climates moist air increases heat loss by improving conduction of heat from the body surface to the atmosphere.

Dry climates therefore cause fewer problems for offshore workers than wet climates.

The body's thermal balance

Your body consists of millions of different types of cells, all of which function best at 98.6°F (37°C). If your body temperature falls below 95°F (35°C) or rises above 105°F (41°C), serious disturbances occur in the cells. If a cold environment causes your body temperature to fall below 95°F (35°C) you will be suffering from hypothermia; while if a hot environment causes your temperature to rise above 105°F (41°C), you will have heat stroke. We shall be discussing both these problems in detail later on in this chapter.

Your cells produce heat, which, to maintain your body temperature at its normal level of 98.6°F (37°C), has to be balanced with the amount of heat your body loses to the surrounding environment. Your body automatically tries to maintain its normal temperature by various mechanisms such as shivering, which are described below.

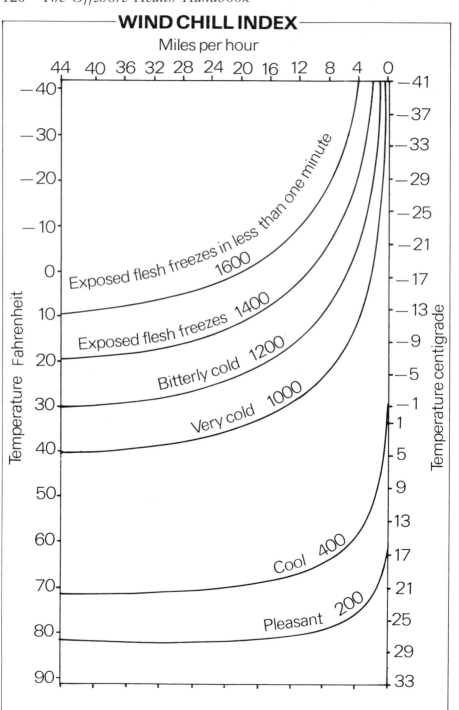

WIND CHILL INDEX

Miles per hour

Exposed flesh freezes in less than one minute 1600

Exposed flesh freezes 1400

Bitterly cold 1200

Very cold 1000

Cool 400

Pleasant 200

How the body gains and loses heat

Heat gain and heat loss from the body to the surrounding environment occur in many ways. The body may take up heat from the radiation of the sun. In a warm climate in full sun, solar radiation can account for 60 per cent of the body's heat gain. It is therefore very important to provide shade for every injured casualty, especially if he is already suffering from heat effects.

The body may gain or lose heat by conduction when it is in contact with another surface. This is much more important in water than in air, because water conducts heat twenty-five times more efficiently than air.

When you stand or walk only a small portion of your body surface is in contact with the hot or cold ground to conduct heat one way or the other. But most casualties will be lying down rather than standing up, so a large area of their body surface will be in contact with the ground, conducting heat to or from the body. Casualties should therefore be insulated from a hot or a cold surface by a poor-conducting material such as clothing.

Body temperature varies around a balance of 37°C according to the interaction of the physiological and environmental factors which help to lose and to gain body heat.

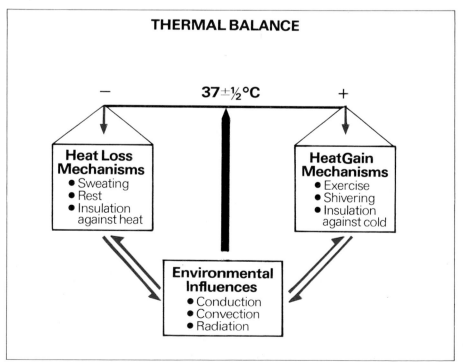

THERMAL BALANCE

$37\pm\frac{1}{2}$°C

—

+

Heat Loss Mechanisms
- Sweating
- Rest
- Insulation against heat

HeatGain Mechanisms
- Exercise
- Shivering
- Insulation against cold

Environmental Influences
- Conduction
- Convection
- Radiation

Effects of cold

Conserving heat in the body
Heat is conserved in the body by insulation and muscular activity.

Insulation   There are many blood vessels in the skin. When your body
has to lose heat the vessels widen, or dilate, so that the blood comes
close to the surface and heat from the blood can radiate away through
the skin. To retain body heat the blood vessels constrict, keeping the
blood away from the skin's surface so the blood heat cannot radiate
away.

As well as this automatic regulation of temperature, layers of insulation, such as clothing or a sleeping bag, will obviously help.

Alcohol should not be given to those suffering from the cold because
it makes the blood vessels near the surface of the skin dilate, resulting
in increased heat loss from radiation.

Muscular activity   If you are working in the open, it is possible to
increase your body's heat production by working harder as the environment cools. The extent to which this is possible depends on your
physical fitness and your ability to sustain a high level of physical
activity. Therefore, as we mentioned earlier in this book, those
employed in cold work-sites must be physically fit.

Shivering very effectively increases your body's heat production by
automatic muscular activity – in fact by 300 per cent over resting
values. This sustained muscular activity is exhausting and because the
muscles require increased quantities of oxygen for energy production
the heart is also put under strain pumping blood to the muscles. This
is an extra reason why no one with a weak or damaged heart should
be employed in a cold offshore environment.

Prevention tips for cold-induced illness

- Do not touch metal with an ungloved hand in temperatures below −68°F
  (−20°C).
- Change wet gloves and socks as urgently as possible.
- Always wear layers of loose clothing which trap air – a poor heat
  conductor.
- Don't forget to protect the head from cold – it is a good heat exchanger.
- Wear well-fitting waterproof boots.
- Watch out for white spots on exposed flesh.
- Beware of loss of sensation in fingers and toes.
- Beware of personality changes in a workmate – the next event may be
  his collapse.

Conditions caused by a cold environment

These may be caused by exposure of one part of the body to cold, such as frostbite or by cooling of the whole body, such as hypothermia. They are all more likely to occur when a cold temperature is associated with high wind speeds.

Cold injuries can be divided into freezing and non-freezing injuries. Of these, chaps and chilblains are examples of minor non-freezing injuries, while trench foot is an example of a serious non-freezing injury. Frostnip and frostbite are, of course, freezing injuries.

Freezing injuries	Non-freezing injuries
• Frostnip	• Trench foot
• Frostbite	• Chilblains
• Cold burn	• Chaps

Frostnip

In very cold conditions, such as those found in Alaska, the Beaufort Sea or the Antarctic, cold injury of exposed parts of the body is a hazard. Frostnip is the first level of this cold injury and is recognized as a white waxy patch usually over the cheek bones or at the tip of the nose. If frostnip is not treated it will destroy the affected tissue and frostbite will result (see next section).

Frostnip and frostbite are not likely to be much of a problem in the maritime environment, but can readily occur if the sea freezes over, in polar and subpolar onshore workings and in a high wind velocity associated with low temperatures. Tissue does not often freeze if the wind-chill factor (see chart on page 128) is less than 1400 (temperature 5 to 14°F or −10 to −15°C).

The time taken for these conditions to develop is variable and depends on the interaction of wind and temperature with the physical fitness, nutritional state and clothing worn by the worker. In severe conditions frostnip can occur in ten to fifteen minutes, and frostbite in an hour or so.

Offshore personnel most likely to be affected are those working outside during drilling, when the wind-chill factor exceeds 1400.

What to do   Frostnip is reversible. Slowly warm the affected area by placing a warm hand (or even a gloved hand) over it until normal colour returns. In polar or subpolar conditions, where frostnip is a particular hazard, personnel should work in pairs and inspect each other's faces and other exposed parts of the body at frequent intervals for its typical white, waxy appearance. Well-fitting adequate dry clothing reduces the likelihood of frostnip occurring.

Recent research (some of it conducted after the 1982 Falklands War) has shown that although frostnip does not result in loss of tissue it sensitizes that area of the body to cold so that future exposure to cold is more likely to produce serious forms of cold injury. This state of sensitization to cold can last for many years after the initial injury and so all offshore personnel working in cold climates must take great care not to sustain such an injury in the first place, by following the preventive advice already given.

Frostbite

This affects exposed parts of the body such as the nose and ears. Frostnip usually occurs first and if it is not recognized and promptly treated frostbite develops, damaging the tissues irreversibly.

In extreme cold, frostbite may also affect the hands and feet. This is much more likely to happen if footwear or gloves become wet, because as we have already pointed out water conducts heat more quickly than air. We cannot stress too strongly that if your feet become wet while working in extreme cold you should stop and change your socks. Good-fitting, non-constricting footwear also helps to prevent frostbite. When gloves become wet the fingertips should be regularly inspected for signs of frostnip until dry gloves can be obtained.

Frostbite can be recognized as a white area on the skin which may be accompanied by blistering. The area will be tender if the frostbite is superficial but numb if the frostbite is deep and the nerve endings have been destroyed. Frostbite ends in gangrene with subsequent loss of the affected area. The aim of treatment is to minimize eventual tissue loss.

What to do   Frostbite should be treated in the following way:

1. Shelter the casualty, give him warm (not hot) drinks if possible, and increase insulation with dry clothing and/or a survival bag.
2. Remove anything tight from the affected area such as gloves or rings because the damaged tissue will swell and they may stop the blood circulation in that area.
3. Take off any wet clothes and cover the frostbitten area with something dry and warm.
4. Thaw the affected area rapidly. This can be done in several ways, depending upon the circumstances:
   - Put the affected area in a lukewarm bath 102–105°F (39–41°C) for 15–50 minutes

- Cover the frostbitten face or ears with a dry gloved hand.
- Place frostbitten hands under the armpits
  - Wrap frostbitten feet in a warm blanket or sleeping bag.
5. Dress the affected area with a light, sterile, non-adherent dressing.
6. Do not rub the affected area.
7. Do not apply direct heat because it can cause burning.
8. Blisters are best left to heal themselves.
9. The casualty needs medical attention.

Cold burn

This thermal injury is caused when metal at very low temperature – usually in an air temperature of −40°F (−40°C) or below – is touched and the skin adheres to the metal. The skin has to be removed from the metal by force as the large mass of metal cannot be rewarmed. Thereafter, the injury should be treated as a burn (see Chapter 4) but should be held under warm running water, around 100°F (40°C), for ten minutes, instead of cold. Remember that sensation may be lost so be careful that the water is not too hot, as this will cause further thermal injury.

The severest cold burn we have seen was sustained at a gas plant during summer in the Arabian Gulf when the liquid nitrogen, used as a coolant had escaped through a faulty flange and rendered adjacent metal extremely cold – even though the air temperature in the sun was 149°F (65°C)!

Chapped hands and lips

Heavy work in a cold, damp environment often leads to chapped, hacked and sore hands and lips. Some people are more susceptible to these than others. A tendency to develop them may be associated with a viral infection. The sore area usually occurs centrally on the lower lip, or at the side of the finger joints. Both of these conditions can cause severe discomfort, and if the hands are badly affected some time off work may be advisable to prevent the condition from deteriorating.

What to do Chapped lips and fingers can be relieved by painting them with Friar's balsam (a resin dissolved in alcohol). The alcohol in the balsam evaporates leaving the resin as a dressing. If this treatment is repeated three times in succession at bedtime, the thick layer of resin excludes the air and healing occurs overnight.

Chilblains

These occur on the fingers and toes following long-term exposure to mild cold temperatures. Young people up to their mid-twenties seem more likely to develop chilblains than older people, although they are not common offshore. Chilblains appear as shiny red areas like mosquito bites which itch. Chilblains usually appear when the living quarters are not properly heated, and usually disappear when the living quarters are adequately heated, no matter how cold the work-site. Most ointments for chilblains are ineffective. There is no need to stop work on account of chilblains.

Trench foot

This condition is rare among offshore workers. It is caused by the combined effects of moderate cold and water on the feet, and usually only occurs if footwear is ill fitting and lets in water. Trench foot varies in severity, but there is usually swelling, redness, pain and numbness in parts of the foot and the best way to prevent it is by wearing well-fitting, water-resistant, dry footwear. If trench foot is recognized early and the feet are dried and warmed they will get better, but if not it can cause continuing pain and discomfort.

Hypothermia

This is not common offshore, and is usually the result of an accident where someone has fallen into the water. Hypothermia occurs when the body temperature falls below 95°F (35°C), normal body temperature being 98.6°F (37°C). When the body begins losing more heat to the surrounding environment than it can produce, the physical mechanisms for maintaining body temperature come into operation. The blood is automatically routed from the surface area of the skin to the internal organs to increase the body's insulation, and shivering begins, which increases the body's warmth by muscle activity. These bodily reflexes may be sufficient to maintain the body temperature, particularly if more clothes are put on and the worker can increase muscle activity by moving faster. But if these reflexes and preventive measures do not maintain the temperature, the body will slowly cool. Eventually a point will be reached when the body's compensatory mechanisms fail and the body temperature falls rapidly until death occurs at any temperature from 91°F (32°C) down to 66°F (18°FC). The features noted at the various temperature levels can be seen in the table opposite.

Body temperature does not fall in an easily predictable way while exposed to cold, which makes it difficult to assess how long someone trapped in the cold is likely to survive.

The management of hypothermia depends on how the condition was caused.

Exposure to dry cold   In this case the temperature falls slowly to dangerous levels and hypothermia is associated with fatigue or exhaus-

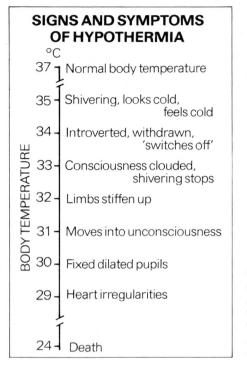

SIGNS AND SYMPTOMS OF HYPOTHERMIA

BODY TEMPERATURE °C

37	Normal body temperature
35	Shivering, looks cold, feels cold
34	Introverted, withdrawn, 'switches off'
33	Consciousness clouded, shivering stops
32	Limbs stiffen up
31	Moves into unconsciousness
30	Fixed dilated pupils
29	Heart irregularities
24	Death

Some of the signs seen as the body cools. The heart is at risk of stopping at any point and is particularly vulnerable when the body temperature reaches 32°C. There is wide variation in the responses of people exposed to cold.

tion. This type of hypothermia is sometimes called exposure or exposure exhaustion. Fatal hypothermia of this type is very rare offshore but it is not uncommon for minor degrees of hypothermia to develop while working in cold weather on the drill floor, or following an accident where a casualty is lying exposed to the elements before being lifted and carried to the sick bay. Because this can adversely affect a man's judgement, it is important to be able to recognize the signs of hypothermia and to know how to treat and prevent it.

The ability of the body to withstand exposure to dry cold depends on:

- Physical fitness
- The environment
- Clothes
- The food available
- Motivation.

Some of these factors can be evaluated when selecting personnel for work in cold areas. Because of the large variability of the above factors,

136 The Offshore Health Handbook

hypothermia can begin to develop while working in a wide range of temperatures. It does not only occur in Arctic regions; in fact, we have attended to one case on midsummer's day in Scotland!

To avoid exposure exhaustion, your clothing and diet should be adequate, and you should take sufficient rests and make an effort to keep warm.

The warning signs of cold exposure are:

- A change of personality: the normally aggressive person becomes withdrawn and apathetic, while the introvert loses his temper and becomes aggressive
- Increasing slowness in physical and mental responses
- Slurring of speech
- Stumbling, cramp and shivering
- Blurred vision.

The supervisor should know his men and be able to recognize these signs and take prompt action.

If any of these symptoms occur in an uninjured man it is essential that he takes shelter and rest immediately. If this is not done the casualty's temperature will fall further and he will collapse from cold exhaustion. He is at risk of dying at any time after his temperature begins to fall below 33°C, but he is unlikely to survive a body temperature lower then 68°F (20°C).

If an injured casualty begins to show signs of cold exposure, do not panic and rush him to shelter before all the necessary first-aid action, such as immobilization of fractures, has been taken (see Chapters 3 and 4). In this situation the casualty's cold exposure should be managed initially on the spot. The correct procedure is:

1. Handle him gently and do not move him unless necessary.
2. Protect him from the wind and rain and insulate him from the wet ground under him.
3. Wrap him in dry clothing, blankets or a sleeping bag.
4. Give him warm drinks.
5. Do not give alcohol.

When the injured or uninjured casualty is eventually returned to the living quarters put him to bed in a warm room. Then report the case to the doctor.

Usually the uninjured victim of cold exposure will feel better after several hours, even before he has reached his normal body temperature. But his judgement may be affected for a day or two, so he should stay in bed for twenty-four hours, and may need to be off work for forty-eight hours, at the doctor's discretion.

Immersion in cold water causes hypothermia to develop more quickly than exposure to dry cold because water conducts heat away from the body more rapidly than air. The symptoms of this type of hypothermia are the same as for cold exposure above.

Divers are particularly susceptible to environmental temperature changes, but being a specialized problem, hypothermia in divers is covered in Chapter 9.

Everyone who falls into the sea experiences some degree of hypothermia, and this happens about once a month in the North Sea. Immersion in cold water may occur following a helicopter ditching (see Chapter 6) or if a man falls overboard from a boat or rig. It is important that the casualty does not struggle or swim vigorously because this will replace the partially warm water trapped in his clothes with cold water which will increase his rate of cooling. To reduce heat loss in the water it is best to remain as immobile as possible. The length of time someone can survive in the sea is extremely variable and depends on many factors. Cases have been reported of people surviving after a day and a half in tropical water, but the average survival time in the North Sea is probably ½–1 hour.

So-called 'post-rescue death' may follow immersion hypothermia. The casualty is successfully recovered from the water (see Chapter 8) and seems to be in a reasonable state of health. A short time later he collapses and dies due to heart failure. This is because immersion in cold water puts a great strain on the heart, as extra oxygen has to be pumped to the muscles. The heart is then put under even more stress when the casualty exerts himself to get out of the water. Another factor is that the pressure of the water assists the return of blood to the heart and this help is suddenly lost when the casualty leaves the water, causing a drop in blood pressure.

The only study into the incidence of post-rescue death was carried out by the Royal Navy, which collected information on survivors of 448 merchant ships sunk during 1940–4. Of 289 people rescued from the water, 160 had been immersed in sea water at 50°F (10°C) or lower. Of them, 17 per cent died within 24 hours of rescue. Of 129 recovered from warmer water, none died suddenly.

The best treatment is to place the casualty in a warm bath 104–106°F (40–42°C) with his arms and legs outside the water so that his body organs are warmed first. It is not necessary to remove the clothes before treatment.

If a bath is not available follow the treatment steps described previously for exposure to dry cold.

Some experts have suggested that giving the casualty warm air to breathe might warm the body organs quickly. In practice this technique does not seem to work because only a very small amount of heat can be passed across the respiratory tract. Only in deep-saturation diving, where helium is breathed, are the lungs important in heat transfer. This is dealt with in Chapter 9.

Effects of heat

It is the summer temperatures in the Arabian Gulf, the Red Sea and the Gulf of Mexico that cause most of the heat-related problems for offshore personnel.

Losing heat from the body
The body has two mechanisms for losing excess heat: reducing insulation and evaporating sweat.

Insulation   The blood vessels in the skin widen, or dilate, allowing heat in the blood to radiate through the skin. The skin becomes pink or red. This automatic reflex can be helped by removing layers of clothing.

Sweating   Sweat glands in the body produce a watery fluid containing small amounts of dissolved substances such as salt (sodium chloride). When the body is hot the glands secrete sweat onto the body surface. The water in the sweat is then very efficiently evaporated using heat from the body. In a very hot climate large amounts of water and salt can be lost from the body in this way and they must be replaced by taking additional salt and drinking plenty of fluids. This sweat-evaporation mechanism can also be mimicked by wetting the body, for example, with a damp sponge, and allowing the body heat to evaporate the water. This is a most effective way of lowering the body temperature.
Whether you can lose heat efficiently depends on your ability to recognize when you are too hot, or whether you are acclimatized to the heat, and on the humidity of the air and the air movement.

Recognizing when you are too hot   People vary in their ability to recognize whether they are too hot or too cold. Those who have difficulty in recognizing whether they are cooling or overheating are less able to shiver and to sweat than the average person. For this reason they often feel that they are physically superior to those who find heat or cold more uncomfortable. In fact they are more vulnerable to heat or cold effects, because they have less warning of the change in temperature than their 'normal' colleagues.

Acclimatization to heat In time the blood vessels near the skin's surface become able to respond more quickly to heat by dilating and allowing body heat to radiate away more rapidly through the skin.

Also very important in the acclimatization to heat is the increasing ability of the sweat glands to produce more and more sweat for evaporation. When fully acclimatized, you sweat very readily and can produce several kilograms of fluid each hour. Acclimatization to heat also results in a reduction in the salt content of the sweat. The newcomer to a hot climate loses less water from sweating, and his sweat contains more salt than the fully acclimatized man.

It usually takes someone from Britain moving to the Arabian Gulf, for example, around two weeks to become acclimatized to the heat. During this time he may suffer from the ill-effects of heat if he is required to carry out much manual work in high temperatures. It is important to be on the look-out for signs of heat exhaustion in these people.

Newcomers to a hot climate should be advised to increase their salt intake as well as their fluid intake, and to undertake only light duties outdoors for the first two weeks. Extra salt intake is best achieved by adding more salt than usual to food rather than taking salt pills. Fruit juices, such as tomato and pineapple juice, should be drunk, as they contain salts in almost ideal concentrations. A good way of replacing the salt lost by sweating is to add one level teaspoon of salt to every 10 pints (5 litres) of drinking water. Such a low concentration is palatable and those who are becoming deprived of salt will find the taste attractive. The amount of fluid that needs to be drunk during hard work in very warm conditions is subject to wide individual variations but can best be judged by keeping an eye on the volume of urine you pass in a twenty-four-hour period. In general this should be approximately 2–3 pints (1–1.5 litres) of a dilute, straw-coloured fluid. If your urine output is less than this and a darker colour, drink more fluids (but not alcohol!).

Humidity The rate of evaporation of sweat into the atmosphere depends on how much water the air already contains. The lower the humidity the easier it is for sweat to be evaporated. That is why it is more comfortable to work in the hot, dry conditions of the Arabian desert than in hot, humid areas at the coast.

Air movement is important in body cooling. The air surrounding the body soon becomes laden with water vapour. Air movement replaces this layer with air containing less water vapour which allows the evaporation of more sweat from the body surface. If the air is still, a casualty suffering from heat effects should be fanned to increase air movement.

What to wear   Temperatures high enough to cook a steak can be tolerated for a period of seconds or even minutes by man without harm, but this depends on the humidity and on his clothing. Much higher temperatures can be tolerated when the skin is covered, and loose clothing, which encourages free circulation of air around the body surface, is preferable. White clothing also reflects the heat and reduces the absorption of radiant heat. The blood vessels of the scalp do not respond to temperature so it is important to protect the head from the heat by wearing a hat, preferably broad-brimmed to help prevent sunburn also (see later in this chapter).

Conditions caused by a hot environment
Heat can produce burns (see pages 86–91). General overheating of the body may cause heat exhaustion or heat stroke. And overexposure to the sun can cause sunburn.

Heat exhaustion
This occurs in conditions hot enough to cause heavy sweating when working hard. It is a disturbance of the body's fluid and salt balance, caused by the secretion of excessive quantities of sweat. It is most common in those not fully acclimatized to the heat, and in accident casualties, but it can also occasionally occur in acclimatized personnel who are working very hard in the heat.
   The onset is slow, around two to three hours, and the following symptoms occur:

- General feeling of weakness and unwellness. The casualty may complain of headaches, dizziness and nausea. He may be restless, lack concentration and be apathetic
- Abdominal cramps
- The body temperature is normal: 98.6°F (37°C)
- The skin is moist and clammy
- Rising pulse and breathing rate.

The fact that the casualty's temperature is normal and his skin wet shows that his body is still able to respond to heat stress by radiating away body heat via dilated blood vessels near the skin's surface and by evaporating sweat. It is most important to treat heat exhaustion, because if it is not treated heat stroke may develop. Heat exhaustion is not a serious condition, but heat stroke can be fatal.

Treatment for heat exhaustion is as follows:

1. Rest the casualty in a shaded, cool area and if outside due to an injury insulate him from the ground – with a blanket, for example.
2. Give him plenty to drink, preferably fruit juice, but if this is not available, give pure water.
3. Do not add salt to the water as a first-aid measure.
4. He must rest for twenty-four hours before he is allowed to work in the heat again.

Heat stroke

This is a serious condition that occurs when the body can no longer control its temperature by sweating. It is not common offshore, except among newcomers to a hot climate, and among casualties who are exposed to the heat following an accident. Unless heat stroke is treated urgently permanent brain damage or death can result. Death usually occurs when the body temperature rises above 113°F (45°C). Heat stroke most commonly occurs following accidents when the casualty is left exposed to the sun.

The onset of heat stroke is usually sudden and it may be preceded by heat exhaustion (see above). The symptoms are:

- Mental confusion and disorientation leading to unconsciousness
- A body temperature greater than 106°F (41°C)
- Hot and dry skin
- Rising pulse rate and noisy breathing.

Treatment is required urgently to reduce the casualty's temperature as quickly as possible.

1. Move him to the shade to protect him from the sun and insulate him from the ground – with a blanket, for example.
2. Wet as much of the body surface as possible with cold or tepid water. This can be done by removing the casualty's clothes and wrapping him in a wet sheet. The water will evaporate, taking heat from the body. Fanning will speed up the rate of cooling.
3. When his temperature has been lowered to normal, 98.4°F (36.9°C), place the casualty in a cool room for twenty-four hours.
4. If the casualty is conscious encourage him to drink as much fluid as possible, either water or fruit juice. This is important, as the heat stroke occurred because his body had run out of available

fluid for sweating.
5. Notify the doctor or rig medic as soon as possible.

Alcohol should never be given to patients with heat stroke, because it dehydrates the body. Salt pills should not be used because they also cause dehydration. Fruit juice contains all the salts necessary, but if fruit juice is not available, pure water provides the best first-aid measure.

Sunburn

People of Celtic ancestry, especially those who are pale skinned and blue eyed, are particularly susceptible to sunburn, which is caused by solar radiation. The burning effects are less marked if exposure is gradual, as this allows time for the protective skin pigment to increase in concentration. These types of people are also very liable to the development of skin cancer following exposure to high concentrations of solar radiation over a number of years.

Sunburn is caused by ultraviolet light and one of the most severe cases of sunburn we have seen was not in a hot climate but in the Antarctic where the ultraviolet rays passed easily through the rarefied, clean atmosphere and where there was intense reflection from the snow surface. Remember that the sea too is an efficient reflector of solar energy.

To prevent sunburn:

- Limit exposure to the sun where possible, especially initially
- Wear a wide-brimmed hat
- Use a sun screen filter preparation, both on exposed skin and under thin clothing.

8. PROBLEMS CAUSED BY WATER, GAS AND NOISE

Water

When a man falls into the water from an offshore installation – as happens around once a month in the North Sea – it is often because he has slipped or had an accidental fall, either from a faulty gangway, or while slung down the side of an installation painting or carrying out repairs. The main problem is to find him and get him out again. In bad conditions, for example in the North Sea where waves may be over 40 ft (12 m) high, rescue is often very difficult. Even with the aid of specially designed standby vessels, fast rescue craft and search-and-rescue helicopters it may take hours to locate the casualty. Although most men succumb to hypothermia after just half an hour in the cold waters of the North Sea, people have been known to survive for over a day in warmer waters (see previous chapter).

Removal from the water
Recovering a conscious man from the water is much easier than removing an unconscious man, who can do nothing to help. The casualty's chances of survival are increased if he can be removed from the water in a horizontal, rather than a vertical position. This is because when he leaves the water the hydrostatic pressure effect of the water on his body is suddenly removed which reduces the blood pressure. If the casualty has hypothermia (see Chapter 7), this may result in sudden and unexpected heart arrest. The horizontal position minimizes this risk by using gravity to help maintain the supply of blood to the brain.

Care and gentleness are essential when removing the casualty from the water. There are well-documented cases of drowning swimmers having their necks broken by the clumsy attempts of rescuers to pull them out of the water. This has resulted in permanent paralysis from the neck down.

Immediate management of the casualty
When a man falls into the water from a ship or an offshore structure and is recovered he may have:

144 The Offshore Health Handbook

- Drowned (see below)
- Injuries, including a head injury (see Chapter 4)
- Hypothermia (see Chapter 7).

Even if the weather conditions are bad the casualty should not be moved until an assessment of his injuries has been made. This is to prevent more damage being caused, for example to an injured spine.

Drowning

Drowning occurs when water prevents oxygen from the air getting to the lungs, and thus to the tissues of the body. The lungs do not fill with water during drowning. Usually, as soon as cold water is breathed in, the upper end of the windpipe goes into a tight spasm, preventing air and water from entering the lungs. The victim may therefore die of drowning, with no water in the lungs at the time of death. If some water is drawn into the lungs it is absorbed into the bloodstream.

Unconscious casualty who is breathing

If the casualty is breathing, you can safely assume that his heart is functioning, even though his pulse is difficult to find. Provided he has sustained no injuries treat him as follows:

1. Protect him from heat or cold.
2. Place him in the recovery position (see pages 45–7) and wait for him to regain consciousness.
3. Seek medical advice and prepare for the casualty to be evacuated to an onshore hospital (see Chapter 6).

This apparently inactive approach is vital. The casualty should not be turned upside down to empty water out of his lungs or stomach. Such action can cause vomiting and stomach contents may then enter the lungs. Clumsy handling of the unconscious casualty may also aggravate an injury.

Unconscious casualty who is not breathing

If breathing cannot be detected:

1. Extend his neck in the same way as for artificial respiration (see page 32). This will prevent the tongue blocking the windpipe.
2. Sweep a finger across the inside of the mouth to remove any obstruction such as a foreign body or a partial dental plate.
3. If breathing is not restored following steps 1 and 2 begin artificial respiration (see page 31). Inflate the lungs by four mouth-to-mouth inhalations in succession.

4. If the carotid pulse can be felt in the neck (see page 37), continue artificial respiration with ten to fourteen breaths per minute until spontaneous breathing is restored.
5. Seek medical advice and prepare for the casualty to be transported to hospital onshore (see Chapter 6).

It may take a long time for normal breathing to return. Therefore continue artificial respiration, because if the casualty's heart is still beating, his chances of survival are high. As with an unconscious casualty who is breathing, attempts to empty water from the lungs are dangerous because they may cause vomiting and they waste precious time.

If the heart is not beating (when the pulse is sought in step 4 above) give external heart compression (see page 35) as well as artificial respiration (see page 31). Continue until breathing and heartbeat are restored or a doctor pronounces the patient dead. Casualties have been successfully revived after several hours of resuscitation so the only reason for stopping it is exhaustion of the resuscitation team, or radioed advice from the onshore doctor.

It is sometimes difficult to be sure whether a casualty is breathing or not, but if there is some doubt little harm will be done by giving artificial respiration. However, serious heart damage can occur if external heart compression is given to a beating heart. For this reason it is vital that all personnel should be able to detect the carotid pulse in the neck (see page 37). The pulse is often difficult to find when the casualty has been immersed in cold water. But if he is still breathing it can be assumed that the heart is still beating.

Secondary drowning
This is caused by the irritant effects of water, mud and sand on the lungs. They disturb the surface lining of the lungs, preventing them from working normally. Secondary drowning can appear from three to forty-eight hours after water has been taken into the lungs. It should be suspected if the casualty develops breathing difficulty within forty-eight hours of inhaling water. All casualties should be sent to hospital as soon as possible after a drowning accident even though they may seem to have recovered. A long period of artificial lung ventilation may be required in an intensive care unit if they have breathing difficulties caused by secondary drowning.

Take medical advice before evacuation, if possible, because there may be a case for giving drugs to minimize the development of secondary drowning.

Gas poisoning

Gassing is a form of poisoning in which the toxic substance enters the body through the lungs. Different gases act in different ways but they all reduce the life-giving supply of oxygen from the lungs to the body's cells. If the casualty is not treated promptly death from lack of oxygen will occur.

How gas poisons the body

Some gases encountered offshore poison by irritating the lining of the lungs, while others interfere with the way the lungs pass oxygen into the bloodstream, yet others act by a combination of these mechanisms. However they act, the end result is failure of oxygen supply to the body cells.

Irritation and inflammation of the lungs may be caused, preventing oxygen entering the body. The irritation may also cause fluid to be exuded from the lungs. A gas which acts in this way is chlorine which is used as a biocide in the processing of oil and for fire-fighting (see later in this chapter). Repeated poisoning with such a gas might result in permanent damage, leading to breathlessness.

Replacement of oxygen   Oxygen is transported in the blood by attaching to red blood cells. Some gases act by becoming attached to the red blood cells instead of oxygen. If these gases are inhaled, oxygen is absorbed through the lung wall but cannot become attached to enough red blood cells and therefore is not transported in sufficient quantities to the body cells. If the body cells do not get enough oxygen, they are damaged and eventually die.

   Carbon monoxide, the poisonous gas in exhaust fumes acts in this way (see later in this chapter). It is attached to the red blood cells 200 times more easily than oxygen, and it gradually accumulates in the blood, preventing oxygen from being transported to the cells. In concentrations as low as ¼ per cent, carbon monoxide can accumulate in this way in the red blood cells. Consciousness is lost when 30 per cent of the red blood cells are carrying carbon monoxide, and breathing usually stops when 70 per cent of the red blood cells have been affected.

   Cyanide gas acts by preventing oxygen from entering the body cells effectively, and is toxic in minute quantities (see later in this chapter).

Irritation and replacement   Some gases, for example hydrogen sulphide, act by a combination of irritation *and* replacement of oxygen. Hydrogen sulphide irritates the eyes even when the gas is present in low concentrations. At high concentrations it may cause fluid to pour out of the lungs causing breathlessness.

But it acts mainly by accumulating gradually in the blood. It occupies space normally used by oxygen when it is transferred from the lungs to the red blood cells. In low concentrations the gas is removed from the blood and converted into a non-toxic substance. As the concentration rises it cannot be removed quickly enough and it accumulates in the blood stopping oxygen reaching the cells. At very high concentrations it causes paralysis of the respiratory centre, preventing breathing, and causing death rapidly.

Treatment for gas poisoning
The general principles of first-aid management are the same regardless of which gas is involved.

1. If you suspect that gas is responsible, sound the alarm before attempting to rescue the casualty. The gas leak may be a sign of a general emergency. If the rescuer is overcome by the gas he will also need help.
2. Before entering the toxic atmosphere put on breathing apparatus. Where possible two people should attempt the rescue together.
3. No matter what injuries are present, remove the patient as quickly as possible from the toxic atmosphere to fresh air.
4. If the casualty is unconscious but his breathing and heart action are satisfactory he should be placed in the recovery position (see page 45) and attended until consciousness returns. When he regains consciousness he should be sent for medical attention.
5. If oxygen is available it should be given to the patient to breathe (see page 58), though fresh air is almost as good. In carbon monoxide poisoning oxygen should be given because it accelerates the removal of the carbon monoxide from the red blood cells (see later in this chapter).
6. If the patient is not breathing give him artificial respiration (see page 31). A mechanical resuscitator should always be used in the case of cyanide poisoning because mouth-to-mouth resuscitation is dangerous for the first aider (see later in this chapter).
7. If the patient's heart has stopped beating give external heart compression (see page 35).
8. When the patient regains consciousness he should be transported to hospital urgently. If lung irritation has occurred it may become gradually worse and require specialist treatment.

In gas poisoning breathing usually stops several minutes before the heart stops. Provided the heart is still beating there is a very good chance that the casualty's life can be saved.

Hydrogen sulphide

This is a colourless gas which is heavier than air. It has a characteristic smell of rotten eggs.

Where it's found   It usually becomes a problem when an oil field has been in operation for some time and water injection is used to flush out the oil after the original pressure in the system has fallen.

It is also found in the openings of pipe lines (pig traps) where a cleaning agent is introduced or removed. It is a major hazard in the offshore workings of the Arabian Gulf and has also been encountered in the recently developed areas of the North Sea.

Hydrogen sulphide may also suddenly be encountered and released during the exploration phase when drilling takes place near gas reserves. It may rapidly envelop the area without warning.

Furthermore, hydrogen sulphide may be produced in stagnant water by sulphate-reducing bacteria. The atmosphere immediately above these stagnant areas of water is dangerous. Stagnant water may accumulate in the legs or bilges of offshore platforms and semisubmersibles, as well as in the oil storage reservoirs and oil–water separators.

Poisonous effects   Opinions vary on the levels of hydrogen sulphide which are dangerous in man. The following is a rough guide:

- 0.1 parts per million   You can smell hydrogen sulphide
- 10 parts per million   You can live with it
- 50 parts per million   Your eyes smart and you cough
- 100 parts per million   You could lose your sense of smell and can die
- 1,000 parts per million   You lose consciousness and can die within a few minutes unless artificial respiration is given at once.

The concentrations of hydrogen sulphide which affect man vary from person to person. In general, this gas irritates the lungs and eyes, damages nervous tissue and accumulates in the blood preventing the transfer of oxygen from the lungs to the red cells.

Loss of the sense of smell at a concentration of approximately 70 parts per million is a danger sign. It is followed by irritation of the eyes and coughing caused by irritation of the throat.

Long-term effects may occur following continual breathing of low levels of hydrogen sulphide (10 parts per million). These include an intolerance to light, an increased secretion of tears and saliva, headaches and dizziness.

Effects on the eyes can be severe following prolonged exposure. There may be intense pain and extreme sensitivity to light. The eyes should be washed out with fresh water following resuscitation from hydrogen sulphide poisoning (see previously).

Prevention All personnel working in areas where hydrogen sulphide exposure may occur (see opposite) should know the procedure to be adopted when there is a leak of the gas. They must also be familiar with the use of the breathing apparatus which has been chosen by their company. Where there is a serious risk of hydrogen sulphide leak it is advisable for special rescue teams to be trained, and for simple mechanical resuscitators to be available. All personnel should be trained to perform artificial respiration. In most cases prompt artificial respiration will save the casualty's life.

Carbon monoxide
Being the toxic gas found in exhaust fumes, carbon monoxide is an ever-present danger offshore. On average we deal with one case of carbon monoxide poisoning every year. Compressors are commonly used on rigs and because they are driven by petrol engines they give off exhaust fumes. A particular hazard is the contamination of air in diving gas when the wind direction allows the exhaust from the compressor to contaminate the air being sucked in at the compressor inlet to the diving gas bottles. This gas is also produced during the combustion of carbon and is therefore associated with fires. It is colourless, odourless and lighter than air. If a man is being rescued from a burning room the rescuer and the casualty should keep as close to the floor as possible, so an appropriate method of lifting which allows this should be chosen (see Chapter 5).

Carbon monoxide is toxic in very low concentrations because it gradually accumulates in the blood. However, a victim overcome by carbon monoxide can be rescued without the rescuer wearing a respirator. This is possible because the rescuer will only be exposed to the gas for a short while, so it will not have time to accumulate in his blood.

Cyanide
This gas is used to disinfect holds and kill rats. It may be found in the holds or bilges of rigs. Very low concentrations of cyanide can be lethal. The chances of surviving cyanide poisoning are very slight. A mechanical resuscitator should be used, since mouth-to-mouth respiration may be dangerous for the first aider.

Using a mechanical resuscitator Portable mechanical resuscitators

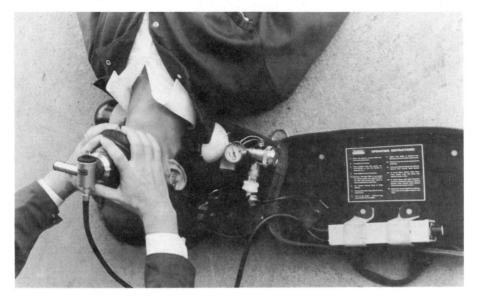

Technique for using a mechanical resuscitator. Open the airway by pulling back gently on the jaw bone. Place the mask firmly against the face for a tight seal.

work from a small oxygen (O_2) cylinder, which will give approximately twenty to thirty minutes use. They differ from the standard oxygen administration equipment described in Chapter 4 by delivering the gas forcefully into the lungs through a seal between the mask and the casualty's mouth. They are normally stored in the sick bay on an offshore installation.

Since the oxygen is stored under pressure, a reducing valve needs to be attached. Connected to this is the patient valve/mask. Before use the O_2 cylinder must be turned on using the key provided. Regular checks of equipment will prevent a cylinder being empty when it is needed in an emergency.

Most resuscitators are automatic and will only need to be set to adult mode. Apply the mask as shown in the illustration, and the rate of breathing and volume will be controlled automatically. Most models are fitted with an obstruction alarm (a loud noise) which indicates an obstruction in the casualty's airway. Appropriate action to clear respiratory obstruction should be carried out, as described in Chapter 3.

There are many different types of resuscitator available, so you must become familiar with how the one on your installation works. But remember that, except for treating poisoning by an extremely toxic gas such as cyanide, efficient mouth-to-mouth respiration (described in

Chapter 3) has a greater chance of success than a badly used mechanical resuscitator.

Nitrogen
This gas is stored in bulk tanks and is used as a blanketing agent for volatile vapours. A leak may therefore replace the air or oxygen in the bulk-tank storage area and cause a man to be faced with a sudden unbreathable atmosphere when he opens the door. The casualty will probably require artificial respiration (see page 31). We deal with around two cases of nitrogen poisoning every five years.

Helium
Poisoning by this gas is about as rare offshore as nitrogen poisoning described above. Helium is used in saturation diving and is stored in cylinder banks on deck. Its main risk is accidental administration to a saturation system without oxygen. If this happens, all the divers in the chamber will suddenly lose consciousness. It is up to the diving supervisor to recognize what has happened and to rectify the balance of gases being delivered to the saturation chamber. Prompt action will restore the divers to consciousness.

Noise

Prolonged exposure to high noise levels over several years causes deafness. This is permanent and not alleviated by conventional hearing aids. But even relatively short periods of exposure can result in

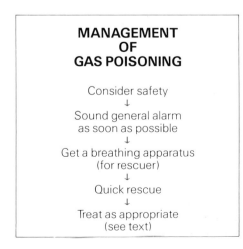

MANAGEMENT
OF
GAS POISONING

Consider safety
↓
Sound general alarm
as soon as possible
↓
Get a breathing apparatus
(for rescuer)
↓
Quick rescue
↓
Treat as appropriate
(see text)

Action flow chart for the management of gas poisoning.

measurable and permanent reductions in hearing ability.

The machinery on an offshore installation can be extremely noisy, particularly in the exploration phase. The offshore worker remains on the installation even when he is not working and the noise of generators and pumps penetrate into the living quarters. This noise may cause stress and prevent sleep. Workers may have to take sedatives at night in order to sleep. This is undesirable because they may become dependent on these drugs. It is also dangerous because in an emergency you have to become instantly awake to prepare for evacuation.

Noise during the day may also be dangerous if it prevents or distorts normal communication, causing mistakes and accidents.

Permissible noise levels

Noise levels for outside work should be maintained below 90 decibels over an eight-hour shift. The noise level should not rise above 70 decibels for workshops and 55 for control rooms. The level in sleeping areas should not exceed 45 decibels.

But in some areas the noise level is unavoidably higher than these recommendations so hearing protection is essential. For example, standard Rolls-Royce turbo-generators are often used in a closed space as a source of power and, despite damping, the noise level may reach 120 decibels. Also, there are often large compressors in the ventilation room. These are used to drive fans and other machinery, the noise level being approximately 120 decibels.

If workers are exposed to a continuous noise level of 90 decibels for 8-hour shifts, then 11 per cent of the work force will eventually develop industrial deafness.

Recommended noise limits on British offshore installations for a 12-hour shift

Area	Noise limit (decibels)
• Workshops	70
• General working areas (outside)	88
• Kitchens	60
• Control rooms	55
• Sleeping areas	45

Controlling noise

Industrial deafness develops insidiously and once it has taken place, little can be done to improve hearing. The effects on hearing depend upon the intensity and type of noise, the duration of exposure, frequency of exposure and intervals between exposure. Prevention of damage to the organ of hearing is vital.

Ear protection must be worn in all noisy working areas. Everyone should be aware of the problems caused by noise and be encouraged to reduce noise as much as possible, for example by shutting doors between noisy areas and the sleeping quarters. The level of noise in various areas of the rig should be monitored at intervals by the employing company to ensure the levels are safe.

9. DIVING PROBLEMS

When an offshore platform is being established, as many diving tasks as possible are performed automatically or by remote control. However, there are still essential tasks which can only be carried out by divers. Following the establishment of the platform there is a continuing need for the underwater section to be inspected regularly by divers. They may also help in repairing any damage.

   If the work is to be done well and with safety the diver must be comfortable and healthy. His concentration must not be disturbed while he is working or manipulating his equipment. Fatigue and breathing nitrogen at depth may affect his judgement. Thermal comfort is also important for divers because they may be distracted by being too hot or cold. Minor changes in body temperature may also affect their judgement or competence.

Diving techniques

The diving technique chosen for a particular task depends on its complexity, the depth of the water and the likely duration of the work.

Free-swimming diver

A free-swimming diver using Self-Contained Underwater Breathing Apparatus (SCUBA) carries his breathing apparatus and gases with him. He has no connection with his surface control. This type of diving is used for work at shallow depths. In the oil industry this type of diving is used in the southern sector of the North Sea, the Mexican Gulf and the Arabian Gulf. In these areas a considerable amount of work can be done at depths not greater than 170 ft (50 m). The commonest problem for SCUBA divers is decompression sickness (see later in this chapter).

Surface supply or bell diving

In this type of diving the diver is lowered to his work-site in a diving bell. The pressure in the bell is increased as he descends to the work-site so that he is breathing gases at the pressure of that simulated depth. He leaves the bell to perform his task then re-enters the bell which is sealed. The bell is then taken to the surface and attached to a pressure chamber. All the while the pressure in the bell is kept the same as that at the work-site. The diver is then decompressed in the relative comfort and safety of a deck decompression chamber. When diving near a complex offshore structure the use of a diving bell greatly increases safety. Diving bells are always used where the depth of the dive is greater than 165 ft (50 m). They are normally used when diving in support of the oil industry in the North Sea.

Bounce diving

A bounce dive is one in which the diver descends to the work-site, performs a task and then returns to the surface. His tissues have usually not had time to equilibrate with the gas pressures at the depth of the work-site.

The time taken for decompression depends on the depth of the dive and the time for which the man remained there. In deep diving therefore, a very short spell of work may require an exceedingly long decompression schedule. This makes bounce diving in deep water dangerous and uneconomical. In order to overcome these problems saturation diving was introduced.

Saturation diving

The point of saturation occurs when all the tissues of the body have become equilibrated with the gases breathed at a particular depth (see pages 160–4). When the diver's body cells have reached the point of saturation with gas they can accept no more. No matter how long he remains at that depth his decompression time will be the same. Therefore, long periods of work can be undertaken with one slow and safe decompression at the end of the work cycle.

In saturation diving the diver remains at the depth of the work-site for his whole work cycle, which may be one, two or three weeks long. At the end of each work shift he is taken from the work-site in a diving bell to a pressure chamber mounted on the deck of the support vessel or structure. He is then maintained at the simulated depth of the work-site until he returns to the job on the next day.

Compression chambers have now become more complex and are known as saturation systems because they consist of a series of interconnecting pressure chambers. Some of these are used for sleeping and others for living accommodation. The atmosphere in the chambers is continuously monitored, and the divers are constantly observed using television cameras. They are cared for throughout their work cycle by highly trained diving supervisors, most of whom are retired divers.

Commercial saturation diving was pioneered during the early 1970s

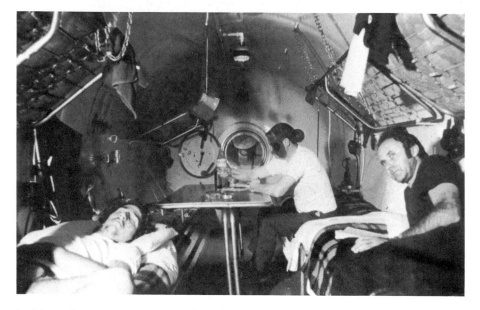

Inside a decompression chamber. Space is limited, even in a large chamber such as this.

in the northern North Sea and it is now the most commonly used technique in that area.

Coping with divers' injuries

When a diver becomes injured or ill he must be removed from the water and put either into a decompression chamber or aboard the vessel which supports his diving activity.

It is not easy to recover an injured diver into a bell and it is extremely difficult if he is unconscious. The problems are caused by the long narrow entrance port, the heavy equipment worn and physical strength required of the co-diver in the hyperbaric environment. These difficulties have been partially overcome by installing a system of pulleys, rather like a block and tackle, inside the rescue bell which can be used to wind the diver into the bell.

When the injured diver has been recovered into the diving bell and the entrance sealed, the time taken to move the bell from the work-site to the deck decompression chamber is generally fifteen to twenty minutes.

The size of the diving bell and the equipment worn by the divers makes it very difficult to perform external heart compression. The best the co-diver can do is to make sure the injured man has a clear airway (see pages 31–2) and is breathing properly. If the casualty is not breathing, artificial respiration (see pages 31–5) should be given if possible. Attempts to compress the heart are not likely to be successful.

In saturation diving the casualty may not be accessible to the doctors for days or weeks because of the long decompression time required. Other injuries such as burst lung and pneumothorax (see pages 167–9), or mediastinal emphysema (see pages 169–70) have to be treated before decompression can begin. In some cases the diver may have reached the surface but has to undergo recompression before the doctor arrives – with cerebral air embolism, for example (see pages 170–1). It is essential therefore that divers should be adequately trained in first aid. Emergency procedures and basic first aid are given in Chapters 3 and 4 of this book, and advice for coping with specific diving-related injuries is included later in this chapter. It is also very important to be able to describe the injured diver's conditions in a way which will be helpful to medical personnel on the rig and onshore (see pages 53–4). They can then give co-divers appropriate instructions for treating the casualty.

Assessing priorities

The commonest mistake when managing an injured diver in a pressure chamber is trying to decompress him too quickly. If there is doubt about what action to take with a casualty it is always best to stop decompression and do nothing until a decision can be taken, with external advice if necessary. A man suffering from pneumothorax will come to no harm unless the pressure is changed. Thoughtlessly continuing the decompression of an injured man may cause additional decompression problems to compound his original injury.

A case which illustrates this point occurred in the mid-1970s in the North Sea when a saturation diver was badly burned by his hot water supply. The attendant was told what treatment to give for the burned area. It was emphasized by the onshore doctor that decompression should be extremely slow because normal decompression tables are designed for healthy divers. The advice was not followed precisely. In order to get the burned patient to medical attention rapidly the decompression was speeded up. The following day the burn had responded to treatment and the patient was very well. But the change in the decompression schedule caused decompression sickness, not in the burned casualty, but in his attendant! The attendant then had to be recompressed and then slowly decompressed. Because of the rapid decompression the attendant had become much more seriously ill than the diver who had been burned.

Diagnosing the injury

A number of devices have been developed over the years to aid diagnosis across the hull of a pressure chamber. It is now possible to take X-ray photographs across the portholes of pressure chambers using portable machines. Flexible X-ray plates have been developed which can be passed through the medical locks of saturation chambers. It is also possible to listen to the chest or the abdomen of a patient using an electric stethoscope which is passed across the hull of a pressure chamber through an electrically insulated penetrator. The doctor tells the diver or co-diver on which part of the body to press the stethoscope so that he can listen from the outside.

A number of other investigations are also possible using suitably insulated penetrators. It is now possible to measure blood pressure, count the pulse rate and even take an electrocardiogram (ECG), showing the patient's heart activity, from outside the pressure chamber. Because of these new developments it is not always necessary for a doctor or nurse to enter the chamber to make a diagnosis. If the co-diver is trained in first aid he should be able to treat the injured diver following instructions from the doctor or specialist at a distance.

Transfer under pressure

Systems have been designed which allow the patient to be transferred from a small offshore chamber to a large operating chamber close to a hospital onshore. The necessary treatment can then be given under close specialist supervision and with the back-up services of the hospital.

A system like this operates for the North Sea region in Aberdeen. It consists of a specially designed titanium capsule which acts as a high-pressure, or hyperbaric, stretcher. It is attached to the offshore pressure chamber and then transferred with the patient to the helicopter. In the helicopter a second chamber with a medical attendant inside has already been compressed to the pressure of the offshore chamber. When the hyperbaric stretcher is attached to the second chamber in the helicopter the doors connecting them are opened and the medical attendant can then help the patient. Both chambers are flown together to the onshore operating chamber and connected to it. The patient and the attendant can then be transferred to the large chamber onshore. The appropriate staff and equipment are already present in the large onshore chamber and are ready to undertake the necessary treatment.

This system has been in existence in Aberdeen for some time. It has been called out on several occasions but at the time of writing has only

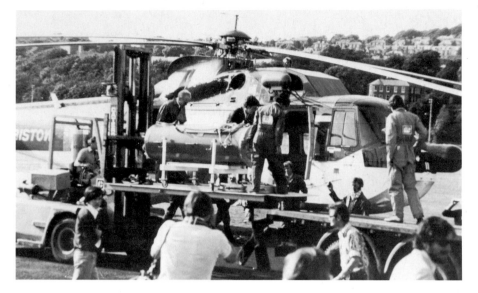

A one-man chamber, the hyperbaric stretcher, being loaded into the helicopter for transport offshore.

The transfer capsule is also loaded onto a helicopter for transport offshore.

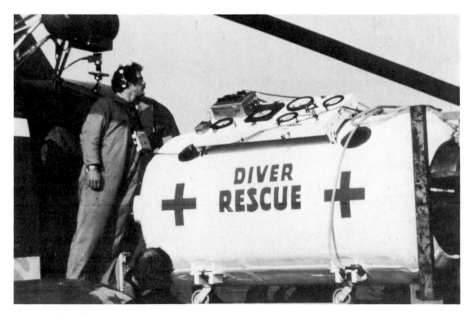

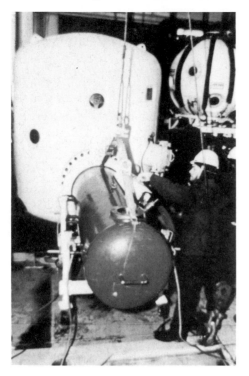

The one-man hyperbaric stretcher is used to evacuate the diver from the commercial chamber. It is then attached to the transfer capsule and taken onshore in the helicopter. The medical attendant inside the transfer capsule has already been compressed to the pressure of the offshore chamber.

been used once. It was used for the management of a patient who sustained a burst lung with mediastinal emphysema at a depth of 400 ft (120 m). After his lung leak had sealed he required a long and slow decompression taking nearly a·month, under careful X-ray control.

Surgical treatment at pressure

In the North Sea there has been no need to undertake surgical treatment at pressure, even though there were two cases of acute appendicitis in the 1970s. Both were treated without operating using gut sedation and antibiotics. Perforated peptic ulcers can also be managed in this way. When acute surgical illness occurs in a remote place it is best to try and treat it without operating.

Changes in the body during diving

Atmospheric pressure

At sea-level the atmosphere exerts a pressure of 14.7 lb on every square inch (1.03 kg on every square centimetre) of the body surface. The surface area of an average man is 18.6 sq ft (1.73 sq m) and the atmosphere exerts 176.6 tons on the surface of his body. He does not feel a great oppressive weight, however, because the gases in the atmosphere enter the air-containing parts of the body, such as the lungs, and come into equilibrium with the body fluids. There is therefore an outward pressure equal to the inward pressure, and they cancel each other out.

Water pressure
Under water there is an increase of pressure because of the column of sea water above the body. This amounts to an extra atmosphere of pressure for every 33 ft (10 m) of sea water. Deep commercial diving in the North Sea usually takes place at a depth of 330–660 ft (100–200 m), at pressures in excess of 11 atmospheres.

Effects of pressure under water
The changes which take place in the body as the diver descends in the water are largely related to the effect of the increasing pressure on the gases he breathes. This is because the volume of a gas is related to the pressure to which it is exposed (Boyle's law). The volume of gas dissolved in a fluid is also related to the pressure of gas to which the fluid is exposed (Henry's law).

The diving values for pressure and depth are regarded as interchangeable; some divers use a pressure value and others a depth value to indicate their position. This table shows the relationship between the values for pressure and depth in common use.

Pressure				Depth	
Atmospheres	Millibars	Psi	Kg/sq cm	Feet sea water	Metres sea water
1	1	14.7	1.03	0	0
2	2	29.4	2.06	33	10
3	3	44.1	3.09	66	20
4	4	58.8	4.12	99	30
5	5	73.5	5.15	132	40
6	6	88.2	6.18	165	50
7	7	102.9	7.21	198	60
8	8	117.6	8.24	231	70
9	9	132.3	9.27	264	80
10	10	147.0	10.33	297	90
11	11	161.7	11.36	330	100

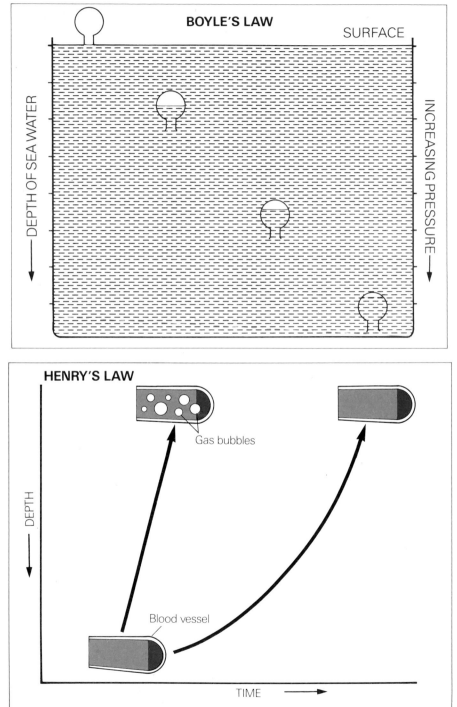

BOYLE'S LAW

SURFACE

DEPTH OF SEA WATER

INCREASING PRESSURE

HENRY'S LAW

DEPTH

Gas bubbles

Blood vessel

TIME

Gases in the body   Pressure changes are considerable in diving. As the diver ascends or descends in the water the volume of the gases contained in the air-containing areas of his body (e.g. lungs, sinuses and ear) varies with depth.

The diver is not normally aware of these volume changes. When the volume of gases contract or expand air passes into or out of his body through the normal passages to make up for the losses or gains.

Sometimes obstructions, such as mucus, develop which prevent the passage of air into or out of the body. This trapped air will then be compressed during diving, and expanded during decompression on returning to the surface. Damage or injury caused by these trapped gases is known as barotrauma or pressure injury (see later in this chapter).

Gases in the blood   As the diver ascends in the water the pressure of the gases in his lungs increases and as he descends it decreases. The quantity of gas dissolved in the blood also increases or decreases in proportion. This takes place immediately but gradually the quantity of gas dissolved in the various fluids within the cells of the body also increases or decreases with depth. The rate at which equilibrium is achieved between the gases dissolved in the blood and the tissues of the body depends on the type of tissue. Because the proportion of the various body tissues (e.g. fat, muscle) is different in different individuals, the time taken to achieve tissue equilibrium, or saturation, varies from one individual to another. The speed and quantity of removal of the gases from the various tissues during decompression or ascent to the surface also varies in different individuals. It is this which makes it difficult to design decompression tables to suit large numbers of people with different body composition.

If the decompression or ascent takes place too rapidly the effect is similar to removing the top off a lemonade bottle too quickly. An excess of the gas suddenly appears from the circulating blood. This may cause an 'air lock' in a blood vessel, cutting off the supply of blood or oxygen to the cells served by that blood vessel. The effect of cutting off the blood to part of the body is decompression sickness (see later in this chapter). The various forms of decompression sickness

Opposite above: Boyle's Law. Water pressure increases with depth and compresses the airspace.

Opposite below: Henry's Law. Approaching the surface too quickly will cause the formation of gas bubbles in the blood vessels as the gas is released from solution. This can be avoided by ensuring the ascent is slow and gradual.

164 The Offshore Health Handbook

are determined by the position in which the block occurs and the tissue which that blood vessel supplies with oxygen.

So, in summary, there are two main forms of illness associated with pressure change:

1. **Barotrauma** is caused by the change in volume of gases with pressure (Boyle's law).
2. **Decompression sickness** is associated with the changing quantities of gas which with pressure become dissolved in the body fluids (Henry's law).

Barotrauma (pressure injury)

Barotrauma occurs when gas in an air-containing part of the body such as the lungs becomes trapped and expands as the diver ascends or contracts as he descends. It may cause damage to organs inside the body because the external pressure squeezes the wall of the air-containing tissue during compression and forces its way through the wall of the tissue during decompression. The danger of barotrauma depends on which body cavity the gas is trapped in. The danger to the diver's life does not always correlate to the amount of pain he suffers. The cavities or tissues of the body which are commonly affected by barotrauma are:

- Middle ear
- Sinuses
- Cavities in decayed teeth
- Lung.

Middle ear
The middle ear is a semiclosed cavity within the ear which is connected to the mouth by a very narrow tube called the Eustachian tube. This often becomes blocked when you have a cold, because the parts of the body around its opening swell. Anyone who has travelled in an aeroplane while suffering from a cold, will have experienced the intense earache which occurs as the pressure and thus the volume of the trapped gas expands when the aeroplane descends to land. The 'popping' of the ears, experienced when descending steep hills rapidly in a motor car, is caused by the gas in the ear expanding and escaping down the tube to the mouth. The ears can be cleared in this way by inducing 'popping'. This can be done by making swallowing movements or chewing movements with the jaw.

Symptoms and treatment If the Eustachian tube becomes blocked during diving, and the ears cannot be cleared the eardrum will rupture, with intense pain. This is unlikely to be fatal but the pain may distract the diver, causing a life-threatening accident. Middle-ear barotrauma occurs rarely in experienced divers who know how to clear their ears. But an upper respiratory infection, such as a cold, causing inflammation around the tube commonly causes the problem to develop unexpectedly. The main symptom is intense pain; blood may also be seen.

The best treatment is to stop compression or decompression until the ears have cleared. The patient should rest and pain-killers can be given. Decongestants may be useful if the blocked tube is caused by a respiratory infection. The patient should not dive again until the infection has cleared up. If his eardrum has ruptured, medical clearance is needed before he can dive again. Healing can take up to six weeks.

The condition sometimes causes perforation of the eardrum in experienced divers going to save the life of a colleague by undertaking rapid compression. Occasionally the drum may rupture without much pain. A perforated eardrum should be suspected if the diver cannot hear well or when blood is seen in the external ear.

Sinus
The sinuses are cavities in the skull just behind the nose. They are connected to the nose by a narrow passage. If this passage becomes blocked, for example when the diver has a cold, air will be trapped in

If the Eustachian tube is blocked, the middle ear becomes a closed air-containing cavity. In diving the eardrum is most at risk. As depth increases, the rising pressure outside the eardrum may cause it to rupture inwards. Conversely, the falling pressure outside the eardrum during ascent may cause the eardrum to rupture outwards.

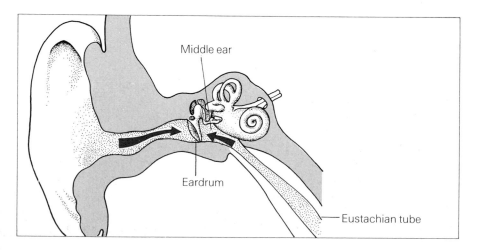

Middle ear

Eardrum

Eustachian tube

the sinuses. As the pressure changes during diving this trapped air causes severe pain in the sinuses. There may also be slight bleeding into the nose or throat. Sinus barotrauma is uncommon in experienced divers.

The best treatment is rest. A pain-killer may be given if necessary. Decongestants may be useful to clear the blocked passages. The casualty should not dive again until the pain has gone and the respiratory infection is cured. Medical attention is not necessary and there will be no long-term damage.

Teeth

If there is a cavity in the tooth, pressure changes may cause the tooth to cave in when the diver descends, or explode when he ascends. Gas spaces at the roots of infected teeth or next to fillings may also cause pain if air is trapped in them under pressure.

Pain-killers can be given and the patient sent for dental treatment. All divers should have regular dental check-ups. Most divers have regular dental examinations and injuries to the teeth caused by pressure are now rare.

Lungs

Barotrauma in the lungs is dangerous and can cause death. Pulmonary barotrauma or burst lung usually occurs suddenly during decompression, often without warning. It can occur at any depth even under small pressure changes.

Pulmonary barotrauma occurs when air is trapped in the lungs during decompression. If the air cannot get out along the normal passage ways when it expands it tears its way through the lung tissue, especially if there is a lung defect. A defect may result from a trivial lung disease or a structural defect with which the diver was born. The diver may have a minor abnormality such as a cyst in the lung which causes no pain. Alternatively he may have a minor lung infection causing secretions which block off a small portion of lung tissue, or he may have asthma, which causes the air passages to narrow.

Medical examination of the lungs is very thorough before a man is allowed to dive, especially if he has had any illness involving the lungs. Because of this scrupulous check-up burst lung is uncommon, with one case occurring every two years in the North Sea in a population of approximately 1,000 divers. Despite its rarity, all divers should become well acquainted with the symptoms and treatment of burst lung — failure to do so could result in the death of a colleague.

There are three types of burst lung, depending on where the air is trapped in the lungs during decompression:

1. Pneumothorax.
2. Mediastinal emphysema.
3. Cerebral arterial air embolism.

Pneumothorax

We see one case of pneumothorax every two or three years. It occurs if the lung bursts on its outer surface, allowing gas to escape into the space between itself and the chest wall.

The diver is usually aware of a sudden sharp pain in his chest and will often become breathless. Further decompression causes the volume of gas trapped between the lung and the chest wall to expand. This collapses the lung and forces the heart against the other lung. The diver then becomes very breathless.

If decompression is not stopped he will die. The air should be removed from the diver's chest by a doctor passing a large hollow needle attached to a non-return valve into the air-containing space and

LEFT: Pneumothorax. A burst lung causes breathlessness and pain. The casualty will die unless decompression is stopped. RIGHT: In tension pneumothorax the casualty's condition will deteriorate even though decompression is stopped. This is because the one way valve created by the burst lung increases pressure within the chest cavity at every breath.

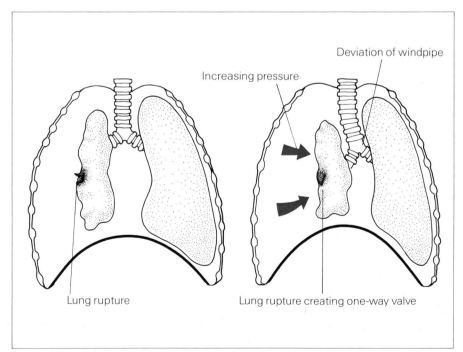

Deviation of windpipe

Increasing pressure

Lung rupture

Lung rupture creating one-way valve

allowing the trapped air to escape through it. A diver with penumo-
thorax in a pressure chamber cannot be decompressed until this has
been done. The diver who has reached the surface before pneumothorax is diagnosed should be treated by chest puncture and not recompressed. Recompression would only be necessary if no doctor were
available to perform the chest puncture and if the casualty were in
acute distress.

Pneumothorax is one of the most serious emergencies in diving. It
should always be suspected when a diver complains of chest pains,
particularly if the pain is accompanied by breathlessness. Decompression should then stop immediately until the cause has been confirmed
by medical diagnosis. Pneumothorax can be diagnosed by taking an
X-ray across the porthole of the pressure chamber and by using an
electric stethoscope. The diagnosis is best made by a doctor who is
then available to carry out treatment.

Provided the casualty is kept at the same pressure he will usually
come to no harm while waiting for the doctor. It is always best for a
doctor to undertake the treatment for pneumorthorax. If the patient
is becoming very breathless he should be placed in a sitting position
which gives the remaining lung tissue maximum oxygen-transferring
capacity. Increasing the pressure of the oxygen breathed should be
done with caution because oxygen poisoning may occur (see later in
this chapter). It may be increased if a patient is suffering severely from
the effects of oxygen lack (he may turn blue or lose consciousness) but
only under the direction of the diving supervisor.

Tension pneumothorax   is an uncommon complication of pneumothorax in which the patient becomes progressively worse even though
the pressure is not changed. This is caused by a flap-like valve at the
point where the lung ruptured which, with each breath, allows more
gas to enter the chest space. This forces the remaining lung further
towards the other side.

Under these emergency circumstances, if no doctor is available, a
suitably trained paramedic should pass an appropriate needle into the
casualty's chest to relieve the air pressure (see illustration opposite).
The paramedic should only carry out this treatment when the patient
is deteriorating and the doctor will not arrive for a long time. If possible
he should communicate with the doctor first.

Long-term effects   Following adequate treatment the pneumothorax
patient should be sent to hospital to recover. He will probably not be
allowed to dive again because his lungs will have been weakened and
there may be adhesions between the lungs and the chest wall. These
would make more diving dangerous.

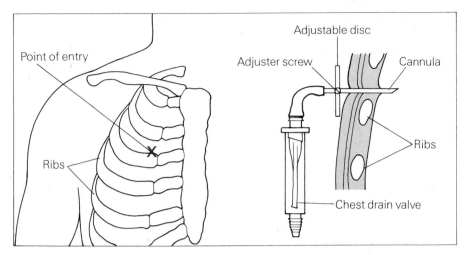

The needle is introduced through the second space between the ribs. It should be just above the third rib, close to the breast bone, and in line with the midpoint of the collar bone. You will feel the tip of the needle entering the chest cavity and see the air escape through the valve.

Pneumothorax
- *Symptoms*
  - Chest pain
  - Breathlessness.
- *Treatment*
  - Stop decompression
  - Call for a doctor
  - When the doctor arrives he will remove the trapped air from the chest space with a hollow needle, once he has made the diagnosis
  - When the trapped air has been removed decompress the patient
  - Send him to hospital.

Mediastinal emphysema
This occurs when the lung bursts during decompression on the side next to the heart and the gullet. Mediastinal emphysema is somewhat more common than pneumothorax; we see around two cases each year. In this condition the lung does not collapse but air from the lung passes into the space between the heart and gullet, known by specialists as the mediastinal area. Properly treated, it resolves readily over a period of up to six weeks.

The symptoms are chest pain and breathlessness. There may be no pain. If the diver is upright the gas in the chest may rise into his neck. It can then be felt as a crackling sensation when the fingers are lightly passed over the neck. If the diver is lying down the gas may pass down his back. The pain caused may be confused with backache or indigestion.

It is important to recognize mediastinal emphysema and to distinguish it from pneumothorax because the treatment is different. If the diver has the symptoms of mediastinal emphysema hold the pressure constant – do not decompress him – and seek medical advice. An X-ray can be taken through the porthole of the pressure chamber and a stethoscope used to listen to his lungs.

If the condition occurs in deep water the patient must be kept at that pressure for several days to allow the lung leak to seal which can only be determined by a doctor. He can then be decompressed very slowly under X-ray control. The bubble of gas in the mediastinal area can be measured on X-ray plates. If decompression takes place too quickly the gas bubble may enlarge. It may then press on the heart or rise into the neck and press on the large blood vessels reducing the oxygen supply to the brain and causing loss of consciousness. Immediate recompression to relieve these symptoms is necessary.

If, however, the diver is decompressed fully and successfully before the diagnosis is made there is little point in recompressing him. It will not help him and may create problems in subsequent decompression. He should be admitted to hospital and kept under observation until the gas has been absorbed into the blood. An investigation of the cause of the barotrauma should be made. Frequently no cause is found but some lung weakness will have occurred and the diver should be advised not to dive again in our opinion.

Mediastinal emphysema
- *Symptoms*
  - Chest pain
  - Breathlessness
  - Crackling sensation in the neck
  - Back pain (occasionally).
- *Treatment*
  - Stop decompression
  - Call the doctor, who will make the diagnosis
  - Do not decompress the patient until the lung leak has sealed (this can take several days)
  - When he is decompressed send him to hospital.

Cerebral arterial air embolism
Along with pneumothorax this is one of the most dire emergencies in diving medicine, being a block of the blood vessels supplying the brain. It is often associated with very fast decompression which occurs when

there is a serious structural failure of the diving system, such as the uncontrolled ascent of a diving bell to the surface when the hatch is open. The condition is uncommon in routine diving.

It is probably caused by the decompression stretching a wide surface area of lung tissue. Consequently small quantities of gas enter the arterial blood circulation to the lungs. These bubbles merge together into larger bubbles, which pass up to the brain in the blood supply, blocking some of the blood vessels in the brain.

When a diver comes to the surface and immediately becomes unconscious cerebral arterial air embolism may be the cause, and should be assumed to be so. The only hope of saving the casualty's life is to get him into a pressure chamber with the best-trained attendant available and recompress him immediately and rapidly to a similated depth of 165 ft (50 m). If he is recompressed and later found not to be suffering from cerebral arterial air embolism no harm will have been done. If the diagnosis was correct, his life may have been saved. When in the pressure chamber he should be managed as any other unconscious casualty (see pages 45–8). He may suffer respiratory and cardiac arrest, so resuscitation may be necessary (see Chapter 3).

The attendant accompanying the patient may suffer a ruptured eardrum because of the rapid recompression. The attendant should therefore not be suffering from any respiratory infections, if possible. Once recompression is completed, the onshore doctor should be contacted, and he will advise on further management.

Cerebral arterial air embolism
- *Symptoms*
  - Blurred vision
  - Chest pain
  - Vertigo
  - Unconsciousness.
- *Treatment*
  - Put the casualty into a pressure chamber with an attendant
  - Recompress him immediately and rapidly to a simulated depth of 165 ft (50 m)
  - Give basic life support as necessary
  - Seek medical advice on a therapeutic decompression.

Preventing barotrauma
1. All those who wish to work in increased atmospheric pressures should have a careful annual medical examination.
2. No one should dive with abnormalities of the lungs, sinuses or ears.

3. No one should dive with a cold or other respiratory infection.
4. Dental hygiene should be carefully maintained. No one should dive with cavities in the teeth.
5. Divers who have sustained injuries to their chest or face should be carefully examined by a doctor before diving again.
6. The diver must be able to clear his ears easily.
7. Barotrauma can be so painful and is so dangerous that if the diver is in any doubt that he is suffering from a condition which might lead to it he should consult a doctor before diving again.

Decompression sickness (The bends)

This is common in SCUBA and bounce diving, but uncommon in saturation diving. It occurs when gas bubbles form in the body fluids during decompression. It is broadly classified into Type 1 (not serious) and Type 2 (potentially lethal) decompression sickness. The various subcategories of decompression sickness are set out in the table below.

Type 1 decompression sickness
Generally Type 1 sickness is not serious, though it may be extremely painful and uncomfortable. It occurs when the blood supply to the muscle, tendon or skin is interrupted by the formation of a gas bubble or 'air lock' in a blood vessel. This is the commonest form of decompression sickness. If it occurs in the skin there may be a skin rash,

Classification of decompression sickness. The type I and type II classification of decompression disorders separate them into 'pain only' and 'serious symptom' categories. This classification – though artificial – has been found to be useful when deciding how to manage a casualty.

Classification of decompression disorders

- Type I   decompression sickness ('pain only')
  - a) Pain *only* in a limb or joint (The bends)
  - b) Itching or swelling of skin

- Type II   decompression sickness ('serious symptom')
  - a) Pulmonary decompression sickness (The chokes)
  - b) Nervous system decompression sickness
    - i) Spinal cord involvement
    - ii) Balance mechanism (The staggers)

swelling, itching and some discomfort. If a limb joint is affected there is usually intense discomfort and pain.

Type 2 decompression sickness

This is a serious form of decompression sickness and if it is left untreated it will probably result in permanent damage such as paralysis or a defect in balance. A gas bubble usually lodges in the lung or nervous tissue. The spinal cord is more readily affected than the brain. The first symptom may be a small area of numbness on a limb. Another common form affects the balance mechanism in the ear and is known as vestibular decompression sickness.

Recognizing decompression sickness

Decompression sickness may be very obvious or appear in a vague way so that even the diver does not suspect it. If it affects the central nervous system the diver's judgement may also be affected. Everyone associated with diving should be able to recognize or at least suspect the condition.

The features of decompression sickness usually relate to the tissue which is involved, and so there may be:

- Severe pain in a limb joint, especially the shoulder
- Breathlessness in lung, or pulmonary, decompression sickness
- Some form of paralysis or sensory disturbance in spinal decompression sickness
- Loss of balance with nausea or vomiting in vestibular decompression sickness.

Symptoms usually appear at least an hour after the decompression has been completed; but they can occur during slow decompression from a deep dive. Because the symptoms are not always clear-cut any unusual complaint or sign occurring within twenty-four hours of a dive should suggest that decompression sickness has occurred. A general feeling of unwellness may be the only symptom.

The minor Type 1 forms of decompression sickness tend to come on earlier and are more common than the serious Type 2 forms. Type 1 symptoms can also mask the early symptoms of serious decompression sickness. The most minor form of decompression sickness must therefore be taken seriously and the casualty carefully observed in case Type 2 decompression sickness develops. Both types of decompression sickness are present concurrently in the same diver in more than 30 per cent of cases.

174   *The Offshore Health Handbook*

Managing decompression sickness
When decompression sickness is diagnosed the correct treatment is to recompress the patient as quickly as possible to the depth at which the symptoms are relieved or to the depth of the original dive. This removes the gas bubble from the circulation. The longer the bubble remains in the blood the more likely that a thick coat of material will form around the bubble; and this layer becomes thicker the longer the bubble is present. If recompression then takes place, the gas may return to solution leaving the solid material in the blood vessel where it will continue to block the circulation.

When time has been allowed for the gas bubble to leave the blood – usually about one hour, the diver should be decompressed following a treatment table, which is slower than usual. There are a variety of treatment tables and many large diving companies use their own. Most authorities use those which have been tried and designed over the years by the British Royal Navy or the US Navy. The choice of table should be made following consultation with a diving doctor.

Decompression sickness
- *Symptoms*
  - Pain in a limb joint
  - Skin rash with swelling and itching
  - Numbness in a small area of a limb of weakness in the legs
  - Loss of balance with nausea and vomiting
  - A general feeling of unwellness
  - Any abnormal symptoms within forty-eight hours of diving.
- *Treatment*
  - Recompress the casualty as quickly as possible
  - Give him fluids to drink
  - When the casualty has recovered he should not be allowed to dive for twelve hours following Type 1 decompression sickness and following Type 2 decompression sickness he should be cleared for diving once again by a doctor.

Effects on divers of gases at pressure

The main gases encountered under pressure are:

- Nitrogen
- Oxygen
- Carbon dioxide
- Helium.

Nitrogen

Nitrogen makes up four-fifths of the earth's atmosphere. It is inert and merely acts as a carrier gas in human breathing, being inhaled into the body with oxygen and exhaled unchanged. Nitrogen makes it impossible to dive with safety deeper than 165 ft (50 m) while breathing air, because at increased pressure it acts like an anaesthetic. At depths as shallow as 100 ft (30 m) it affects performance in the same way as a small quantity of alcohol. The effect, called nitrogen narcosis, becomes progressively more marked as depth increases. Susceptibility to nitrogen narcosis varies from person to person, but at depths greater than 165 ft (50 m) the effects are dangerous. Commercial air diving is normally restricted to this depth for this reason.

Nitrogen narcosis, like drunkenness, is characterized by euphoria, sleepiness, lack of concentration and impaired coordination. If a diver notices these feelings he should rapidly lessen his depth. Unfortunately the overconfidence which comes with drinking alcohol also occurs with nitrogen narcosis.

The co-diver may not experience nitrogen narcosis at the same depth as his partner. If a diver sees signs of unusual action in his co-diver he should suspect nitrogen narcosis, particularly if they are diving at approximately 165 ft (50 m), and make sure his partner reduces his depth.

Nitrogen narcosis
- *Symptoms*
  - Same as the effects of alcohol
  - Euphoria
  - Lack of concentration and coordination.
- *Treatment*
  - Reduce the diving depth.

Oxygen

A lack or excess of oxygen results in serious problems to the cells of the body.

Hypoxia or lack of oxygen may occur if there is a low percentage of oxygen in the air cylinder or an inadequate flow rate. It may also occur following an accident, if the airline breaks, for example.

The casualty may appear blue and be breathless, or may become unconscious. If he is unconscious treat him as described on page 45.

Pulmonary oxygen poisoning (lungs) may occur in divers given oxygen to breathe at pressures greater than 0.5 atmosphere absolute and less than 3 atmospheres absolute for a continuous period of 15 or 16 hours or an intermittent period of exposure lasting a few hours at a time over several days.

In order to prevent this excessive quantity of oxygen being delivered to the tissue cells and damaging them the lung walls become thickened to reduce the rate at which they transfer oxygen to the body's cells. The lung walls readily return to normal when the oxygen pressure is reduced, but repeated episodes of pulmonary oxygen poisoning can cause permanent damage to the lungs. The oxygen pressure in a diving gas mixture is usually kept well below 0.5 atmosphere of oxygen and pulmonary oxygen poisoning is therefore uncommon. But it can occur if high-pressure oxygen is used to treat decompression sickness.

The symptoms are irritation of the throat leading to coughing, a sharp nagging pain behind the breastbone and an increased rate of breathing. The toxicity of the oxygen depends on the partial pressure of the oxygen, the duration of exposure and the diver's susceptibility.

The only treatment is to reduce the amount of oxygen breathed in.

Neurological oxygen poisoning (brain) may occur when pure oxygen is breathed at high concentrations under a pressure equivalent to that at 100 ft (30 m) depth. This may occur when a breathing set is charged with pure oxygen. It does not occur often in saturation diving but may occur in bounce diving and when decompression schedules are used. Neurological oxygen poisoning is most likely to occur in a pressure chamber during decompression. But it may also develop during treatment with oxygen at increased pressure, for instance when treating decompression sickness.

Neurological oxygen poisoning affects the brain. It may cause a convulsion like an epileptic fit. There is wide-ranging susceptibility between divers, and the susceptibility of the same diver can also vary from day to day. The main danger is that the casualty may injure himself by falling on the ground. There are few warning symptoms, although a major convulsion may be preceded by a sensation like pins and needles or by twitching of the lips.

The oxygen pressure must be reduced immediately and the sufferer prevented from injuring himself (see how to manage an epileptic fit on pages 48–9). Basically this can be done by keeping him quiet and still. There are no residual effects provided the pressure of oxygen is reduced straight away. Neurological oxygen poisoning can be prevented if the divers are not given oxygen to breathe at a pressure greater than 2.5 atmospheres absolute.

Carbon dioxide
In saturation diving systems the environment is monitored very precisely so that the temperature, the oxygen pressure and the carbon

dioxide pressure are all maintained at the correct levels. The carbon
dioxide exhaled by the diver is removed by passing the chamber gas
over soda lime, which absorbs the carbon dioxide. The level is
constantly monitored to ensure that this scrubbing mechanism is
performed correctly. Divers spend a great part of their life breathing
various gas mixtures through long and complicated systems of tubes.
Because of this they may be exposed to slightly increased concentrations of carbon dioxide. Very experienced divers may be more
tolerant to an increase in carbon dioxide pressure than the new diver.
But some people are abnormally sensitive to carbon dioxide and this
may be the cause of some unexplained cases of unconsciousness in new
divers.

At normal pressure, carbon dioxide poisoning occurs if concentration rises above 4 per cent. In diving it may happen if the scrubbing
system is not working efficiently, or if there is inadequate ventilation
or contamination of the breathing gases.

The first symptoms are a throbbing headache, dizziness and confusion. The diver will be flushed, sweating and breathing deeply. Eventually he will become unconscious.

He should be removed from the carbon dioxide atmosphere as soon
as possible and treated for unconsciousness (see page 45). Artificial
respiration (see page 31) should be given if breathing has ceased, and
until the brain recovers.

To prevent carbon dioxide poisoning, the diving system should be
adequately ventilated, and continually and properly monitored to
measure the gas present.

Helium

For many years diving was restricted to 165 ft (50 m) because nitrogen
narcosis occurred at deeper levels. The search for an alternative gas to
mix with the oxygen and dilute it to suitable levels for breathing led
to the use of helium. Helium is not narcotic at the pressures used in
saturation diving; but it is scarce and expensive. Continuing research
has not found a cheaper alternative, though hydrogen is currently being
examined.

The main problems associated with helium are the high pressure
neurological syndrome (HPNS), voice distortion and temperature
control. In addition, helium poisoning can occur if pure helium is
delivered to the divers in error; this problem is covered in Chapter 8.

HPNS may occur when breathing a helium mixture at depths greater
than 500 ft (150 m). The diver becomes dizzy, he may have tremors,
find it hard to breathe and have difficulty swallowing. He will eventually become unconscious. HPNS may be reduced by adding some

nitrogen to the helium mixture and reducing the speed of compression. At the time of writing, though, this technique is still the subject of research.

When the symptoms occur in a diver not much can be done since he is separated from his attendants by a wall of steel, and reduction of pressure at great depth may take several days.

Voice distortion   The density of helium is so different from that of nitrogen that it causes voice distortion. This may cause problems when monitoring the diver in the water, assessing his requirements and understanding his problems. It also creates difficulties when managing illness because communications are difficult. Unscramblers are available for helium speech and are improving year by year, but they are still not perfect. So it is important that divers speak precisely and their supervisors learn to understand them readily. Learning to lip read may help. It is important not to try and complete an unfinished sentence for the diver. He may not be trying to say what is expected. Errors like this may cause serious mistakes in the management of an emergency. For this reason, and because the communication may pass through several hands before it reaches the diving medical advisor, important messages should always be written as well as spoken.

Temperature control is a problem when breathing helium because of its high thermal conductivity. This means that as a diver goes deeper and the gas he breathes becomes more and more dense it becomes a better conductor of heat. The heat loss from his respiratory tract eventually becomes very great. At a depth of 1,000 ft (300 m) all the heat produced by the body is lost through the respiratory tract. At that depth the diver loses heat at a rate related to the temperature of his surrounding environment and its density. With no gas temperature control this would not give him long to live in very cold water. When he is in the saturation system the gases he breathes are maintained at a precise temperature level. And when he is in the water, heat is added externally to his body by means of a hot-water suit. These measures counteract the loss of heat from the respiratory tract. At depths greater than 500 ft (150 m) some additional form of heating is necessary to maintain thermal balance. This is usually provided by adding a heat exchanger to the gas supply.

It has never been proved, but it seems very likely that many of the diving accidents in the North Sea in the latter part of the 1970s were related to inadequate diver heating. Divers may not be able to determine whether their body temperature is too hot or too cold, which can lead to dangerous mistakes as minor degrees of cooling or heating may affect judgement and competence (for treatment see discussion of hypothermia in Chapter 7).

Divers are vulnerable to environmental temperature because of the increased density of the gases which surround them and which they breathe. They are therefore liable to overheating if the environmental temperature is high or overcooling if it is low. It is the diving supervisor's responsibility to maintain optimum environmental temperatures for his divers.

Other diving problems

Drowning
See page 144.

Ear infections

In saturation environments the harmless bacteria which normally live in the human ear cannot survive. When they have died, other more harmful organisms, such as the bacteria *Pseudomonas pyocyaneus* and *Escherichia coli* can enter the ear and cause infection.

When a diver carrying *Pseudomonas* in his ear enters a pressure chamber the whole team is likely to become infected in four to five days. If none of the divers is carrying the germ in his ear then the condition may not appear for about fourteen days (he may be carrying it in other parts of his body). For this reason some diving companies take swabs of the ears of the divers before allowing them to begin a saturation dive which is intended to last for a long time.

The symptoms of infection are severe pain in the ears and this may be associated with vertigo. The pain may be so bad that the dive has to be aborted.

These infections can be minimized if:

- The pressure chamber is kept clean and the humidity is kept as low as possible.
- Divers maintain scrupulous personal hygiene
- Divers use protective ear drops (5 per cent aluminium acetate).

If the diver is in pain he can be given pain-killers. He will always improve when he returns to normal atmospheric conditions. The ear should be swabbed, and the swab sent ashore for identification of the germ responsible and advice on the possible use of antibiotics.

In normal conditions the untreated germ may persist in the ear without causing any trouble for as long as six weeks following decompression, after the symptoms have subsided. As soon as the diver is saturated the germs multiply and the infection begins again.

Other ear infections can occur in the cells lining the ear if they become soggy and water-logged. In many cases yeasts are responsible for the infections. The main symptoms are severe swelling in the ear with pain and redness.

Treatment is by giving pain-killers and antiseptic drops, such as 5 per cent aluminium acetate drops.

Avoiding contamination of the diver's environment

It is important not to contaminate the divers' breathing system or pressure chamber with toxic materials. Compressors and filters should be maintained carefully so that machine lubricating oil does not enter the breathing gases.

Epoxy resins have recently been introduced as a means of repairing concrete underwater structures. Great care must be taken to avoid introducing these substances into a pressure chamber because they would contaminate the atmosphere.

10. INFECTIONS OFFSHORE

Living quarters on offshore rigs are often overcrowded. In these circumstances infections may pass readily from one man to another. Inadequate standards of personal hygiene and poor hygiene in the preparation and storage of food will aid this process. Water must also be monitored carefully for contamination; and it may have to be purified before it is drunk.

It is important for all offshore personnel to be aware of the factors which can lead to infections, to be able to recognize the symptoms and to know what action to take should infection break out. A widespread outbreak of infection could temporarily close a platform, and would be dangerous for the workers affected and the adjacent onshore communities, where patients may be evacuated.

Food poisoning

This only occurs if food or water is contaminated with certain germs. It can be passed from one man to another by poor hygiene, such as not washing your hands after using the toilet. There is also variation in the susceptibility of individuals – some people becoming ill after eating contaminated food, while others remain unaffected.

Much can be done to prevent food poisoning by careful preparation, handling and storage of food.

Effects of temperature on germs

Germs in food multiply rapidly when they are kept at 50–140°F (10–60°C). They begin to die at temperatures above 150°F (65°C), depending on how long they are kept at the high temperature. Below 50°F (10°C) many germs survive though they may not multiply at that temperature. The organism causing typhoid fever, for example, is killed by heat, but is extremely resistant to cold.

It is also important to note that some germs produce poisons which are not destroyed by heat. If foods containing such germs have been left lying exposed for long enough before cooking, they can be very dangerous to eat even after full cooking.

Frozen foods These should be stored carefully in properly sealed containers. A separate defrosting area should be set aside and used for nothing else. It is very dangerous if cooked meats are allowed to come into contact with the defrosting liquids from poultry. The germs in the poultry will be destroyed by thorough cooking after it has defrosted but the contaminated cooked meat will not be heated again and therefore any dangerous organisms present in the defrosting liquids will not be killed.

The ideal temperature for defrosting is 50°F (10°C) and it should never be higher. Defrosting should never be speeded up by immersing the frozen food in hot water or by direct heat. Microwave defrosting is safe, provided the maker's instructions are followed precisely. All meat should be free of frost particles before cooking. Once meat has been thawed it should only be refrozen if it has been cooked since thawing.

High-risk foods

Trifles, cream cakes, custards and sauces provide ideal areas for the growth of germs. Particularly as these types of food are often left over from one meal to another and allowed to stand in the open.

Fish Especially shellfish, is very liable to contain harmful organisms even when fresh and before it has been cooked. Special care should be taken not to store cooked fish dishes, especially when the fish is mixed with food like rice or mayonnaise.

Meat and poultry should never be left standing in a warm atmosphere. This applies to raw, as well as cooked meat. Poultry must be completely defrosted before cooking. If meat dishes are prepared before they are required, they should be:

1. Chilled as quickly as possible after cooking and stored in a refrigerator.
2. Thoroughly reheated when they are required for eating.
3. Dishes such as shepherd's pie must be thoroughly re-cooked rather than just reheated.

Storing food
- Only food needed for immediate use should be kept in the kitchen
- Food must be stored in clean, cool areas and in suitable containers
- The containers must be cleaned and sterilized or disinfected regularly. Sterilization is carried out by boiling the container.

Containers may be disinfected by using a proprietary solution
- Cooked and uncooked foods should not be stored together
- There should be separate refrigerators for cooked and uncooked foods
- Food should not be kept in the refrigerator for more than a few days
- Regular inspection must be made for pests which carry disease, such as mice and cockroaches
- Suitable containers must be provided for kitchen waste which are sealable and vermin proof
- Bins should be washed and sterilized with boiling water each time they are emptied.

Water
Water is probably a greater source of disease than food in isolated, remote communities such as oil and gas rigs. It is usually in short supply and often has to be brought to the site or prepared so that it is fit for human consumption.

Water fit for drinking should be:

- Free from visible suspended matter, colour, odour and taste
- Free from bacteria and disease-causing organisms
- Free of mineral or organic matter which is dangerous to health.

Making water fit to drink   Suspended matter can be removed from water by filtration. Water can be sterilized in several ways. Usually specially prepared solutions of sodium hypochlorite containing not less than 10 per cent by weight of available chlorine are used. The sodium hypochlorite is thoroughly mixed with the water so that a slight excess of free chlorine is present in the water after a contact period of not less than 30 minutes. The dose is 1–5 parts of sodium hypochlorite per million parts of water (300 ml sodium hypochlorite solution to 500 litres water). When the chlorine has been in contact with the water for 30 minutes sodium thiosulphate granules or pills are added to the water to remove the excess chlorine and make the water palatable.

Non-bacterial food poisoning
In offshore work-sites, which contain a variety of chemicals, such as drilling mud and phenols to treat waxy crude oil, it is important to remember that chemical contamination of food or water can cause illness. Hands and face should be washed before eating and contaminated outer work-clothes and boots should be taken off before entering the living and eating quarters.

Personal hygiene for food handlers

These standards below are the minimum which must be strictly adhered to if the work force is to be kept safe in a closed community.

- Take a bath or shower daily
- Wear clean protective clothing at all times
- All cuts and sores should be shown to the rig medic and covered by a clean waterproof dressing
- Food handlers with infected sores should not be allowed to work in the kitchen
- Nails to be kept short and fingers clean
- No smoking in the kitchen
- Always wash hands after using the toilet
- Always avoid touching hair or mouth while preparing food
- Even minor tummy upsets to be reported to the medic
- All outdoor clothing to be kept outside the kitchen.

Kitchens are warm and moist, and provide ideal conditions for the multiplication of germs, so scrupulous hygiene must be maintained by all kitchen staff.

Kitchen cleanliness

Kitchen cleaning routines should be laid down and carried out by personnel not involved in cooking.

- Floors should be washed daily
- Tables and worktops should be regularly washed and disinfected once a day
- Staff toilets must be cleaned and disinfected once a day, nail brushes must be supplied and a notice provided to remind food handlers to wash their hands after using the toilet
- Machinery coming into contact with food must be washed daily and equipment coming into contact with high risk food should also be stripped and sterilized with boiling water each day.

Recognizing and treating food poisoning

The symptoms of food poisoning are vomiting and diarrhoea, with cramping or griping abdominal pain. These are symptoms of the way the body attempts to get rid of the poisonous material as fast as possible. In general the sooner the symptoms appear after an infected meal the more severe the food poisoning. Usually several people are affected.

Depending on the germ responsible, food poisoning can involve just a minor episode of diarrhoea and vomiting, or be a life-threatening condition. The appearance of shock (see page 54) is a sign of infection by a dangerous germ, and indicates that there is a serious problem which needs urgent medical help, as many people may be infected.

A large amount of fluid can be lost through vomit and diarrhoea and the casualty must drink enough to replace these losses. If possible the victims should be isolated and have their own toilet facilities, as germs can be spread through the faeces. If this is not possible, hygiene procedures must be very strict. In fact, medical advice should always be sought, even for minor episodes.

Action following a severe outbreak of food poisoning
1. Inform medical officer ashore.
2. Isolate patients.
3. Take specimens of vomit and faeces for analysis onshore.
4. Close the catering facility.
5. Find out how many people have severe and mild symptoms.
6. Attempt to identify the food causing the outbreak of poisoning by interviewing the victims.

Other infections found offshore

The normal shift system of two to three weeks on duty followed by two to three weeks ashore means that personnel can return to the offshore structure incubating a disease. Thus, it is possible for all communicable diseases to appear offshore, where they can be spread rapidly in the confined environment of the rig.

Workers from other countries, particularly those from Third World countries, may introduce diseases uncommon in the host country, such as malaria and amoebic dysentery.

Treatment
If any infectious diseases such as hepatitis or measles are suspected the patient should be isolated and given separate hygiene facilities until help is available or he is no longer infectious. Most germs can be transmitted through the faeces, the blood or the breath. In the absence of a rig medic, the onshore doctor's advice should be sought if someone offshore is suspected of having contracted an infectious disease.

Normally, anyone with symptoms of an infectious disease which could threaten the smooth running of an offshore installation will be brought back onshore. In Britain the evacuation should be coordinated by the environmental health adviser, whose job is to liaise between the installation and the public health authorities onshore (see Chapter 2).

Vulnerability

When a group of men live closely together for several months in the remote, isolated environment of an offshore installation their resistance to germs may decrease. These workers may be particularly vulnerable to infection when they next come into contact with a new series of germs brought onto the rig by the next group of people to arrive.

Infestations

Head lice

These are becoming more common. They affect all types of people, are not associated with dirty heads, and are easily transmitted from one head to another. They cannot hop or jump but are passed on from one person to another by head to head contact.

Head lice are flat-backed insects a little smaller than a match head. They are greyish-white in colour and are found on hair and the skin of the head, especially behind the ears and the back of the neck. Head lice live for approximately one month and feed off blood they take from the scalp. Away from the head they die within forty-eight hours. The female head louse lays approximately 270–300 eggs during her lifetime. The eggs (nits) are the size of a pin-head, white and oval and they may be mistaken for dandruff.

The eggs are 'cemented' near the hair roots and cannot be removed using ordinary combs. They hatch within 7–10 days.

Signs of head lice are itching of the scalp, restlessness and general malaise. Infection of the scalp may result.

Lotions and shampoos based on modern insecticides such as malathion and carbaryl are effective against head lice. They kill the lice and their eggs on contact. Prioderm, carylderm and quellada are suitable products which can be used in lotion or shampoo form.

Treatment with Prioderm and Carylderm lotions (see 'pubic lice' for treatment with Quellada lotion):
1. Rub the lotion into the scalp and other infected areas of the body and leave for twenty-four hours. Both preparations should kill eggs and lice in one application.
2. Do not apply the lotion to wet hair. Do not use artificial heat on the hair because it may degrade the insecticide. Both preparations also contain alcohol which is inflammable. Do not allow the hair to come into contact with chlorine.
3. Comb out the lice with a very fine-toothed comb. When the eggs are dead they turn a red or black colour.
4. Have regular checks with the rig medic or doctor.

Treatment with Prioderm, Carylderm and Quellada shampoos is the same as above though the shampoos are applied to wet hair, massaged in and left for four minutes. The hair is then rinsed, shampooed in the normal way, rinsed, dried and combed. If a second application is necessary give it on the following day.

Pubic or crab lice
These lice are spread via sexual intercourse and any close physical contact (but rarely through clothing, bedding or toilet seats). The main symptom is itching.

Treatment with Quellada shampoo
1. Put two tablespoons of the shampoo on the affected area and any adjacent hairy areas. Do not get the shampoo near the eyes.
2. Rub the shampoo in vigorously for at least four minutes.
3. Wet the affected area thoroughly with warm water and work the shampoo into a lather.
4. Rinse thoroughly, rub with a clean dry towel.
5. Use a fine-toothed comb to remove the lice.
6. If the lice are not all removed repeat the treatment after twenty-four hours but do not use the treatment more than twice a week.
7. Put on clean clothes and launder others. Use clean bed linen.

Treatment with Quellada lotion
1. Apply the lotion to the affected area and any surrounding hairy areas.
2. Leave the lotion on the area for twelve to twenty-four hours.
3. Wash it off thoroughly.
4. Put on clean clothes and launder others. Use clean bed linen.
5. A second application is not usually required but if it is needed apply it four days after the first treatment.

Scabies
Scabies is a skin disease caused by common mites which burrow under the skin. It is easily spread by contact with an infected person. Scabies causes intense itching, soreness and inflammation of the skin. It generally occurs on the fingers, hands, chest, underarm area, waist, groin, buttocks, knees and ankles. It will not affect your ability to work.

Treatment with Quellada lotion
1. Apply a thin layer of lotion to the whole body except for the face and scalp. If any parts of the body are not covered with the lotion the treatment may not be successful. Do not get lotion in the eyes.

2. Leave it on the skin for twenty-four hours then wash thoroughly.
3. Put on clean clothes and launder others. Use clean bed linen.

Athlete's foot
Athlete's foot is a fungal infection of the foot. The symptom is itching of the feet. The area between the toes can crack causing the skin to peel off. It is very easily spread, especially in warm, damp areas. It will not affect your ability to work.

1. Wash the feet regularly and dry them well. Then apply an anti-fungal powder (e.g. Mycil) thoroughly on the feet and between the toes.
2. Shoes may have to be treated as well.
3. Each person should use his own towel which is washed immediately after use.
4. Don't walk around in bare feet as this encourages the spread of infection.

EPILOGUE

The technological advances made in the past decade by the oil and gas industry have been truly amazing and the indications are that progress continues as deeper and deeper waters are explored in more and more remote parts of the earth. The current exploration of the Beaufort Sea in the high Arctic testifies to this and undoubtedly the resources around the great continental mass of Antarctica will eventually be tapped. This will probably not require a greatly different system of health care, but there will be a need for even more intensive preparation and training, together with the provision of more sophisticated communication equipment if the same required high standard of health care is to be maintained.

In this book we have tried to impart all the information you need if you work or plan to work offshore—or in any other remote place—today, and you wish to ensure a high standard of health care for yourself and for those with whom you work. But there is no substitute for practical experience, especially when learning emergency techniques. This type of experience as well as more theoretical knowledge can be obtained at the various offshore training centres, a list of which we have included overleaf.

USEFUL ADDRESSES

BRITAIN

Aberdeen Industrial Doctors
24 Albyn Place
Aberdeen
Contact: Mrs M. MacRae,
Company Administrator
Telephone: (0224) 572879
Telex: 739148 Sharet G

Centre for Offshore Health
RGIT
Kepplestone Mansion
Viewfield Road
Aberdeen AB9 2PF
Contact: Prof J. N. Norman,
Director
Telephone: (0224) 33866
Telex: 739148 Sharet G

Centre for Offshore Survival
RGIT
352 King Street
Aberdeen
Contact: Mr J. H. Cross,
Director
Telephone: (0224) 638970
Telex: 739212

Occupational Health Ltd
North Sea Hyperbaric Centre
Howemoss Drive
Kirkhill Industrial Estate
Dyce
Aberdeen

Contact: Dr C. M. Childs,
Director
Telephone: (0224) 770987
Telex: 739272 IUC SCO G

Offshore Medical Support
12 Sunnybank Road
Aberdeen
Contact: Mr D. Webster,
General Manager
Telephone: (0224) 492884
Telex: 73677 Casvac G

**Institute of Environmental and
Offshore Medicine**
University of Aberdeen
Ashgrove Road West
Aberdeen
Contact: Mr D. Webster,
Business Adviser
Telephone: (0224) 681818
Telex: 73458 Uniabn G

North Sea Medical Centre
Lowestoft Road
Gorleston-on-Sea
Great Yarmouth
Norfolk, NR31 6QB
Contact: Mr J. S. Dick,
General Manager
Telephone: (0493) 663264
Telex: 975118 NORMED G

British Antarctic Survey
High Cross
Madingley Road
Cambridge, CB3 0ET

Contact: Dr R. M. Laws,
Director
Telephone: (0223) 61188
Telex: 817725 BASCAM G

Society of Underwater
Technology
1 Birdcage Walk,
London, SW14 9J5

Contact: The Chairman
Telephone: (01) 222 8658
Telex: 917944

Institute of Petroleum
61 New Cavendish Street
London, W1M 8AR

Contact: Mr D. Payne,
General Secretary
Telephone: (01) 636 1004
Telex: 264380

Health & Safety Executive
25 Chapel Street
London NW1 5DT

Contact: Dr J. T. Carter
Director of Medical
Services
Telephone: (01) 262 3277
Telex: 299950

AUSTRALIA

Department of Service and
Technology
Antarctic Division
Channel Highway
Kingston
Tasmania 7150

Contact: The Director
Telephone: 29 0209
Telex: AA 57090

ACKNOWLEDGEMENTS

We gratefully acknowledge the wise counsel of Mr I. W. B. Johnson, Senior Training Officer at the Centre for Offshore Health for his useful criticisms and discussions. We would like to thank Mr D. W. Chrystal and Dr S. E. Wilcock of the Centre for their valuable advice and to Mrs A. Jones, Mrs C. Taylor and Miss H. Rennie for undertaking the bulk of the typing with great patience and forebearance.

We also acknowledge, with many thanks, the help and encouragement received from Mr J. H. Cross, Director of the Offshore Survival Centre, RGIT; Dr Z. Abu Risheh, Chief Medical Officer of the Combined ADMA–OPCO and ADCO Medical Services, Abu Dhabi; Dr A. M. House, Director of the Centre for Offshore and Remote Medicine, Memorial University of Newfoundland, Canada and Dr W. L. B. Leese, Consultant to the Centre for Offshore Health, RGIT.

Finally, we specially wish to acknowledge all the encouragement and enthusiastic support we have received in the development of our subject from Professor Blyth McNaughton, Head of the School of Mechanical and Offshore Engineering at RGIT and from Dr Peter Clarke, Principal of RGIT.

Prof J. Nelson Norman and John A. Brebner 1985

The publishers would like to acknowledge the following individuals and organizations for their help during the preparation of this book: Messrs K. Mills, R. Morton and G. Page for providing the clinical pictures on pages 64, 65, 76, 77, 88 and 93; Mobil North Sea, London for photograph on pages 9, 120; Dr R. M. Hastings for taking most of the remaining photographs with considerable expertise and Mr W. Black for processing the films.

The diagrams and cover design were drawn by David Gifford.

INDEX

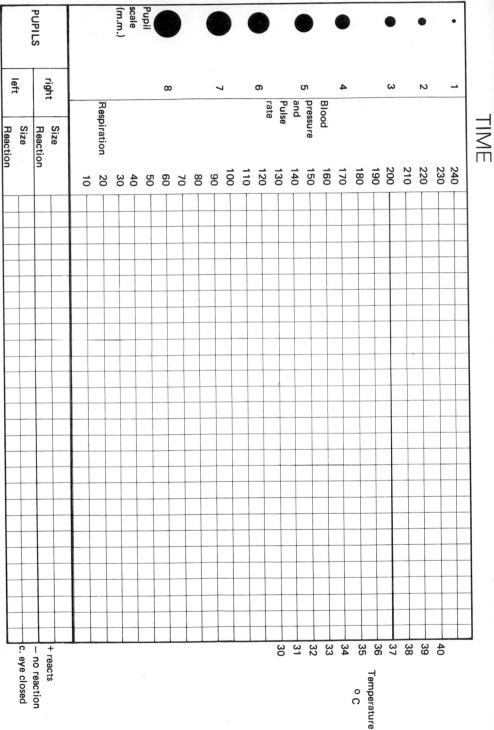

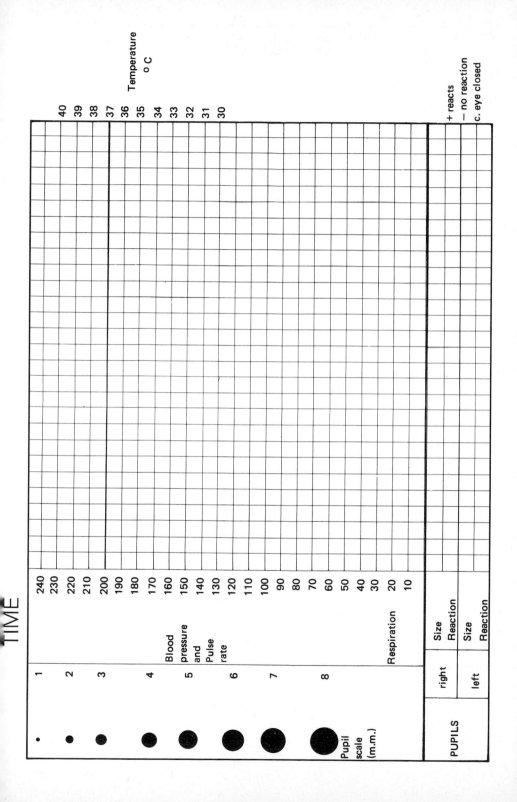

TIME

PUPILS	right	Size
		Reaction
	left	Size
		Reaction

Pupil scale (m.m.)

1
2
3
4
5
6
7
8

Blood pressure and Pulse rate

240
230
220
210
200
190
180
170
160
150
140
130
120
110
100
90
80
70
60
50
40
30
20
10

Respiration

Temperature °C

40
39
38
37
36
35
34
33
32
31
30

+ reacts
− no reaction
c. eye closed

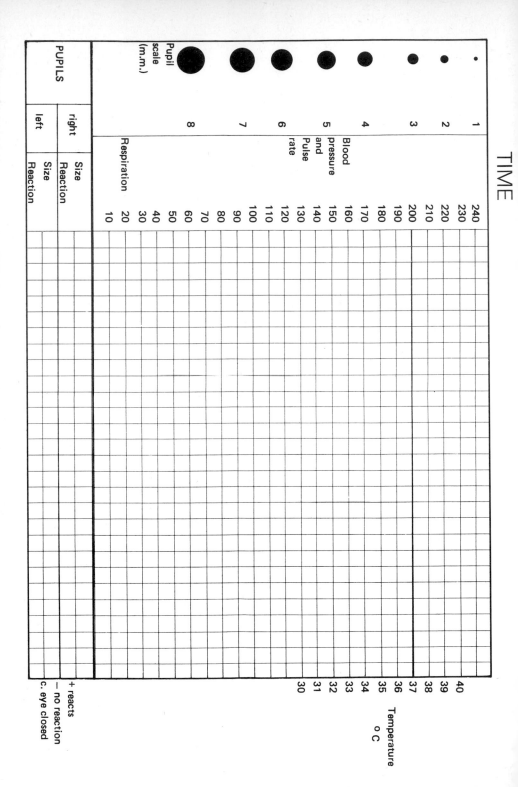

The Practical Problems in Medicine Series
(for medical professionals)

PRACTICAL PROBLEMS IN DERMATOLOGY
Ronald Marks, Professor of Dermatology, Welsh National School of Medicine.

PRACTICAL PROBLEMS IN RHEUMATOLOGY
Frank Dudley Hart, Consultant Physician, Westminster Hospital.

PSYCHIATRY: COMMON DRUG TREATMENTS
Roy Spector, Professor of Applied Pharmacology, Guy's Hospital. Medical School; **Howard Rogers**, Professor of Clinical Pharmacology, Guy's Hospital Medical School and Consultant Physician, Guy's Hospital; **David Roy**, Consultant Psychiatrist, Goodmayes Hospital, and Senior Lecturer in Psychiatry, St Bartholomew's Hospital.

PRACTICAL MANAGEMENT OF ASTHMA
Tim Clark, Professor of Thoracic Medicine at Guy's Hospital Medical School and **John Rees**, Consultant Physician at Guy's and Lewisham Hospitals.